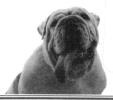

Is Your Dog a Chow Hound in the Making?

Consider some of the biggest mistakes people make when it comes to their dogs' diet, exercise, and health habits:

✔ Do you feed your dog a commercial food? If so, it's likely that the food has rewired your dog's natural appetite, making him eat more than he needs even when he isn't hungry.

✔ Do you feed your dog treats? Those seemingly innocent treats can actually addict your dog to sugar, salt, and fat.

✔ Is your dog a carboholic? Many commercial foods contain too many carbohydrates, setting your dog on a course to pack on the pounds.

✔ Do you feed your dog as the label recommends? If so, you're probably overfeeding your dog every day.

✔ Is your dog a couch potato or lap lump? Many dog owners have disrupted their dogs' metabolism by not exercising them enough.

✔ Do you think your dog is just fluffy, not fat? Then you may be stuck in the fat gap, having forgotten what a normal-weight dog looks like.

Whether we know it or not, we're partially to blame for encouraging an unhealthy lifestyle for our dogs. But don't worry, *Chow Hounds* gives you the skinny on keeping your dog healthy and provides simple solutions for shedding the excess weight.

Chow HOUNDS

Why Our Dogs Are Getting Fatter
and a Vet's Plan to Save Their Lives

Ernie Ward, DVM

Health Communications, Inc.
Deerfield Beach, Florida

www.hcibooks.com

To my wife, Laura, for her unwavering love,

belief in me, and significant contributions to this book;

to my parents for filling my childhood with pets.

Library of Congress Cataloging-in-Publication Data

Ward, Ernie.
    Chow hounds : why our dogs are getting fatter : a vet's plan to save their lives / Ernie Ward.
      p. cm.
    Includes bibliographical references and index.
    ISBN 978-0-7573-1366-0
    1. Dogs—Diseases—Diet therapy. 2. Dogs—Health. 3. Dogs—Food—Recipes. 4. Obesity in animals. I. Title.
    SF991.W37 2010
    636.7'089325—dc22

                         2009052246

Publisher: Health Communications, Inc.
          3201 S.W. 15th Street
          Deerfield Beach, FL 33442–8190

Cover photos ©2009 Inmagine
Cover design by Larissa Hise Henoch
Interior design and formatting by Lawna Patterson Oldfield

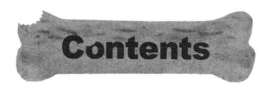

Contents

v

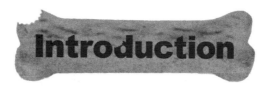

Introduction

WE'RE KILLING OUR DOGS BY MAKING THEM FAT.
There, I've said it. That single observation led me to write this book.
As a practicing veterinarian for almost twenty years, I was witnessing
the gradual deterioration of our pets' health on a daily basis. My patients
were getting fatter and facing more debilitating diseases as a result. The
frightening fact was that no one was discussing it. The question was,
"Why not?"

The answer, as you'll discover in reading this book, is complicated.
From how veterinarians are taught and practice nutrition to manipu-
lation on the part of pet-food manufacturers, from our society's insatiable urge to include food into every act of life to a subtle shift in
what we perceive as normal weight—all of these factors and more
have created an epidemic of obese pets. And it's killing our pets. Sadly,
we're raising the first generation of dogs that likely won't live as long
as their parents.

This is a troubling paradox since we love our four-legged family
members more than ever. Over the course of my lifetime, I've witnessed
dogs going from backyards to our bedrooms, from kennels to couches,
from the bedroom floor to sharing a pillow. I've even known wives
who kicked their husbands out of bed because their dog "needed more
space" or "couldn't deal with the snoring."

Yet just as dogs are becoming part of our extended families, their waistlines have also been expanding. Almost half of America's best friends are now overweight, a number that has been increasing for the past decade. And with this extra weight comes a greater risk for crippling arthritis, respiratory disease, and lives cut short. The good news is that I have devised a prescriptive plan that can restore almost any dog back to health, often in less than six months. I have used this plan successfully for many canine cases and with human patients—beginning with my own health crisis.

Bettering Health in Pets and People

When I was in veterinary school, I received one of those dreaded calls that no one wants to get: My father had been rushed to the intensive care unit of a hospital for open heart surgery. He was only forty-eight. Sure, my dad had put on a few pounds recently, but so had everyone. I grew up in the deep-fried South and accepted a potbelly as a rite of passage. A strong southern man, his left coronary artery had become blocked, compliments of a lifelong diet replete with fried foods and rich desserts. My family and I were terrified. If this could happen to him, it could happen to any of us. That was when I stopped eating meat and fried foods.

In the ten years that followed, my father's health improved. I continued being a "mostly-vegetarian" (I still ate fish occasionally), and I figured I was doing as much as anyone to stave off heart disease. *Vegetarians don't get heart disease,* I thought. The problem was, I was a junk-food vegetarian.

Junk-food vegetarians are more common than you might guess. While they don't eat meat, they eat lots of carbohydrates, fats, and sugars—not to mention processed soy and processed anything that doesn't include meat, poultry, pork, or fish. This "fake-healthy" regimen took its toll. As I approached thirty, I was just over 5'7" and weighed 165 pounds. But I couldn't jog a mile without my knees screaming, and my idea of stress release was drinking two or three beers. Always on edge, I began to dread the long hours of veterinary practice and I had a short temper with my wife.

Like other successful and crazy-busy professionals, I had allowed my physical well-being to take a back seat to my career. The trouble with this "work-only" approach is that I didn't have time for the most important things in life: my spouse, family, health, and creative pursuits. The better I was becoming as a doctor, the worse I felt. On the eve of my thirtieth birthday, I looked in the mirror and saw a pale, bloated, sallow-faced man. On that day, I made a commitment to change my life—and I did. By age forty, I was regularly completing long-course triathlons, including the Ironman, and I had a stronger relationship with my wife and my children.

As I changed myself, I began changing my veterinary practice. In veterinary school, I'd been taught how to treat diseases, not prevent them. No one taught me to view food as medicine or how nutrition could preserve health. Most of the veterinary nutritional training I received was driven by pet food companies. So, I began to fill in the gaps in my understanding of veterinary nutrition. Wanting to share my knowledge, every client received nutritional and exercise recommendations during their exam. The results were staggering.

The more I embraced a holistic, nutrition, and lifestyle-based approach, the better my patients responded. Dogs that once could barely stand were soon able to walk around the block; patients with cancer lived longer than expected; diabetic pets no longer needed insulin injections; and my human clients reconnected with their best friends.

After seeing how powerful these lifestyle changes could be, I declared war on excess weight and vowed to discuss the diet and lifestyle of pets with anyone willing to listen. I had seen how exercise and food transformed my life and my patients' health, and I wanted to share this information with everyone.

In 2005 I founded the Association for Pet Obesity Prevention to reverse the deadly trend of pet obesity by opening people's eyes to the truth about their pets' health. The last few decades have created a perfect storm for portly pets, and it's difficult for owners to reverse the tide. What many dog owners don't know is that many of the "healthy" dog foods they are buying are so spiked with sugar and fat that they have actually changed their dogs' brain chemistry and addicted them to overeat. Compounding the problem, pet food labels are often difficult for consumers to interpret, and therefore they rely on word-of-mouth recommendations from pet stores, breeders, and veterinarians, many of whom know little beyond the dog food company's flashy brochures. This book will help you see beyond the hype and take control of your dog's health. It is filled with the latest science, some real case examples, and simple-to-implement diet and exercise regimens. The information will challenge many of your beliefs and shed light on the importance of keeping your dog lean. In short, this book may not only help your dog live a longer, healthier life, it may very well *save* your dog's life.

Shelby's Health Makeover

SHELBY, A FIVE-YEAR-OLD LABRADOR, had always been "big boned." Her owners brought her in because she was having trouble getting up after lying down and she struggled to climb into the car. The owners suspected a hip or knee sprain. They were a bit surprised when I told them the cause of Shelby's problem was her weight, not a sprain; that premature arthritis was causing her lameness.

Shelby was young. In fact, in human terms she was about as old as her owners. They didn't feel arthritic and couldn't believe Shelby was any different.

X-rays confirmed my suspicions. Both knees and hips demonstrated evidence of early osteoarthritis. Supplements and medications could ease Shelby's pain. That was the easy part.

The harder part was changing Shelby's lifestyle—more specifically, how her pet parents cared for her. Despite the owner's opinion, Shelby's overeating wasn't due to a problem with Shelby but with the owners. They had a deep-seated belief that Shelby had always been a "big girl." As I explained that weight loss only offered the chance to slow down the progression of the arthritis, I had my doubts that the owners would change their ways. Thousands of cases had taught me not to expect every client to heed my recommendations. Success with my patients had less to do with what I prescribed than what the owners did.

Complicating matters was the fact that Shelby's owners were obese, which always makes my job a little more challenging: telling obese clients that their dog is obese. I've learned to be sensitive and polite, while persuasive and direct.

As I continued outlining my plan for Shelby, I witnessed one of those rare moments of insight and clarity: They got it. They were really listening. Within one month Shelby had lost 5 pounds. At four months, she was 18 pounds lighter, more muscled, and feeling spry. Her owners exclaimed that Shelby was jumping into the car and meeting them at the door each morning for their walk.

At our six month recheck, I noticed that Shelby wasn't the only one losing weight. Both of Shelby's owners informed me that they had lost fifteen of the 55 pounds they were going to lose. They even challenged me to run with them in a 5K the upcoming spring, which we all completed together.

Shelby continues to be a patient of mine, and I couldn't be prouder of the family. After five years of struggling to have children, they recently welcomed their first. Shelby continues to be the matron of the family, caring for not only the two-legged child but the family's new four-legged one as well. Shelby's knees and hips are surprisingly healthy, benefiting from decreased weight, daily exercise, and nutritional supplements.

If you're reading this book, I know you care for your pet. You're reading this book because you want your dog to have the best possible quality of life. Even if your pet is currently overweight or obese, you can change your pet's life for the better. Within your hands, you have the power to make changes that will help your pet live longer, develop fewer diseases, and increase the likelihood of aging with vigor and grace the way nature intended.

Your dog can achieve Shelby's success . . . with your help.

1

PET OBESITY:
A Supersized Problem

PET OBESITY IS A HUGE PROBLEM. How big? To better answer this question, the Association for Pet Obesity Prevention (APOP), conducted the first National Pet Obesity Awareness Day Study in 2007. The findings were alarming: 43 percent of all dogs were assessed by a veterinary health-care provider as overweight or obese. By 2009, the findings were worse: 45 percent of all dogs—almost one-half—were classified as overweight or obese. And what if your dog isn't obese but is just toting around a few extra pounds? Owners who view their dogs' "few extra pounds" as no big deal are greatly underestimating the potential health threat. Even as few as two or three extra pounds may be silently damaging your dog's vital organs.

> **❝ Owners who view their dogs' 'few extra pounds' as no big deal are greatly underestimating the potential health threat. Even as few as two or three extra pounds may be silently damaging your dog's vital organs. ❞**

The Problem with Extra Pounds

When I was in veterinary school in the late 1980s, very little emphasis was placed on the role fat tissue played in maintaining health or causing disease, especially in dogs and cats. In all honesty, fat was viewed as an inert by-product of excess calories. Unfortunately, that way of thinking hasn't changed much even though numerous studies have now proven that fat is a much more active tissue than we ever imagined and a direct cause of a multitude of diseases. These findings have led scientists to refer to fat as the "second pancreas" because of the number of hormones and compounds that fat tissue secretes.

 EYE ON THE SCIENCE

Anatomy of a Fat Cell

THE MAJORITY OF FAT CELLS are created during the early stages of growth, especially the first four to six months of life in dogs. Puppies that gain weight rapidly and become overweight during this period produce large numbers of fat cells (a type of hyperplasia) that will remain with them throughout their lives, predisposing them to obesity. In adult dogs, the majority of weight gain is due to enlargement of the preexisting fat cells, called *hypertrophy*. Unfortunately, recent research demonstrates that adult animals can produce new fat cells, especially when they are obese. A study published in the October 2004 edition of the journal of the Federation of American Societies for Experimental Biology found a possible mechanism for obese mice to create additional new fat cells. Perhaps of greater concern was the researcher's warning that childhood obesity seems to predispose adults to obesity, even if they lose weight during adolescence and early adulthood. In mice, the connection seems apparent. My years of clinical experience with dogs indicate that pudgy puppies become obese adults.

All fat is not created equal. There are two types of fat: white adipose tissue and brown adipose tissue, which serve two different purposes and behave very differently in the body. White adipose tissue is the most common type of fatty tissue found in dogs and humans. Historically, white adipose tissue was thought to serve three primary functions: heat insulation, cushioning of vital organs, and, most important, as being a source of energy. We now know about a dark side to excess fat. Current scientific thought places a danger sign clearly above increased abdominal or belly fat—the fat you may see hanging down on your dog's underside just behind the ribs. In humans, this area is known affectionately as a potbelly and results from too much white adipose tissue. Researchers have discovered that this belly fat produces a multitude of chemicals and compounds that signal other cells to perform some action. Some of these actions are beneficial, while others are potentially damaging and can cause conditions such as high blood pressure and diabetes. Because excess fat produces harmful molecules, obese dogs are in a chronically inflamed state, akin to having an endless infection or fever. In fact, in an article in *Science*, researchers at Boston's Dana-Farber Cancer Institute characterized obesity as a "low-grade inflammatory state" that was unhealthy and contributed to a number of medical problems.

Why Addressing Canine Obesity Is Important

1. **You want your dog to live a long time.** Overweight pets, like people, have a higher incidence of life-stealing health complications.
2. **You want your dog to be healthy and active.** Dogs were meant to run and play. Obesity robs them of the ability to enjoy and lead an active life.
3. **You want your dog to be pain-free and happy.** One of the main complications of obesity is painful arthritis. Your dog deserves a pain-free life.
4. **You want your dog to live a life without medications.** All medications carry risk. If you can avoid drugs, you should.
5. **You want to save money on your pet's bills.** Obesity complications are expensive. The surest way to save money is to prevent disease.

From "The Promise" to Potato Nation: The Evolution of Couch Potatoes and Lap Lumps

To understand the reasons our pets are fatter now, we must go back in time to when humans and dogs first roamed the planet together. Many pet lovers think of their pets as their babies or as family members. From an emotional perspective, I couldn't agree more. From a physiological perspective, dogs are maybe not quite family, but more like really strange-looking cousins. Dogs and humans share more physiological and digestive similarities than cats and people, or cats and dogs.

Depending on which research you accept, humans have been sharing their lives with dogs for somewhere between 35,000 and 85,000 years. One of the key reasons humans and dogs began to hang out together was that we share a common diet; food fueled our bond. Another key reason was that we both are excellent persistence hunters. That is, we both possess similar endurance and tracking abilities, and we work well together.

For thousands of years, dogs lived primarily off food scraps we offered and food they foraged themselves. Few other animals are as well-suited for this type of collaboration with humans. From our complementary senses to our nutrient requirements to our intelligence, dogs and humans are perfectly paired. I daresay humans wouldn't be where we are today without our trusty canines. As we evolved together, we became increasingly interdependent on each other. In this way we developed what I call The Promise. The Promise refers to the fact that dogs, by using their heightened sense of smell and hearing, would aid us in obtaining food and warn us of approaching danger. For humans, The Promise is to protect our dogs from stronger predators; provide them with food, water, and shelter; and nourish their young. Our love affair with dogs is rooted in The Promise and exists even today. Instead of hunting and guarding, dogs today mostly provide compassion and companionship. The trouble is we've taken The Promise too far in terms of providing food and shelter and are now inadvertently harming our beloved companions.

Ten thousand years ago, or even 100 years ago, life was very different. Most people grew their own food, made their own clothes, and built their own houses. Today, these jobs are outsourced, which is not necessarily a positive development from a health perspective. Americans are less active than ever before. According to the Nielsen Company, the average American watches more than four hours of TV every day. That adds up to twenty-eight hours a week or two months each year spent virtually still in front of a screen. If a person lives to sixty-five years of age, that person will have spent nine years glued to the tube. You don't have to be a genius to calculate that we're not moving much. And if we're not moving, neither are our pets.

Even worse, many dog owners don't walk their dog beyond the distance required for bathroom duties. If this sounds eerily similar to the human obesity epidemic, we've got thousands of years of cohabitation to blame. Our dogs have adopted our lifestyles and have consequently inherited our problems. In an effort to make our lives easier, we've only served to make our lives and the lives of our dogs less healthy.

Shrinking Spaces and Expanding Waists

According to the National Multi Housing Council, 15 percent of Americans live in rented apartments, opting to occupy condominiums or duplexes for convenience (no yard work!) and cost. This downsizing affects our dogs. Apartment living means less backyard to walk or play in. Many people don't walk their dogs around the block because they're concerned how their dog will behave or react to strangers. But the problem exists in suburbia, too.

The Fallacy of Fences

Many dog owners are mistakenly under the impression that if they have a backyard, their dog will get plenty of exercise. Open the door in the morning, let the dog out, and it will run to its heart's content. Not true.

Who wants to run around all by themselves? Dogs are pack creatures; they like to do things in packs. Put a dog alone outside and watch what happens. First, they'll run around the borders of the yard checking for intruders. Most dog owners witness this and somehow assume this must be what goes on forever. "You should see him when I open the door. He takes off like a madman!" After a few minutes without discovering any intruders, the dog settles down. Instinctively, dogs seek to conserve energy (just like their human companions). Without a reason to do otherwise, most dogs find a comfy place to lie down until something interesting happens. Usually it doesn't.

After some time, the dog's owner opens the door and all he sees is his dog charging for the door. "Wow, that dog never slows down!" he muses. He missed the entire "lying down, doing nothing" part. As soon as his dog detects the door is about to open, *bam!* he's off like a rocket. If you don't believe me, try this simple experiment. Before putting your dog outside in the morning, take a video camera and place it so you can film most of your backyard. Turn it on and return inside. Let your dog out as you would normally. Videotape for ten to twenty minutes. Review tape. Weep.

Roaming in Black-and-White

Remember Jeff Miller and his dog Lassie of the hit 1950s television show *Lassie*? Lassie, an exceptionally gifted collie, helped the son of a war widow deal with the pressure of growing up on a weathered old farm in rural America. Along the way, Lassie helps prevent a variety of catastrophes, save numerous lives, and catch a couple of burglars.

The television show *Lassie* wouldn't be made today. It's too unrealistic for present-day society. Video games have replaced outdoor activities. Playing with the dog is way down on the list after text messaging. Lassie and the ideals of outdoor physical fun have been left behind in the world of black-and-white. High-definition virtual reality is slowly but surely replacing the real world just beyond our doors.

While we can't go back and revisit the days of black-and-white living, we can do as much as we can to care for and nourish our pets. When we don't, we all pay the price in poor health, stress, and decreased quality of life. For most of us, living requires spending time with our pets; anything less leaves us empty and incomplete. This book will help you maximize the time you spend with you pet, beginning with becoming a more informed consumer when it comes the food that you're feeding your dog.

2

MARKETING ADDICTION:
The Epidemic of Kibble Crack

MAYBE YOU'VE WITNESSED THIS: As you approach your refrigerator, your dog runs up and begins barking and wagging her tail excitedly. Perhaps when you reach for a box of your dog's favorite treats, she begins to act puppylike and appears ecstatic. Maybe you even have a dog with super hearing: regardless of where your dog may be in your house, as soon as you pour her food, she appears from nowhere. If you've observed any of these behaviors, you're not alone. This typical doggy dinner display means that dog food manufacturers have succeeded in their jobs. They have tweaked their foods to the point that they have manipulated your dog's appetite, making him addicted to overeating. In truth, many dog foods and treats are the equivalent of "Kibble Crack," addicting our nation's dogs to added fat and sugar. By cleverly manipulating food labels and ingredient lists and selling you a false sense of fulfillment, pet food companies have literally changed your attitude and your dog's behavior toward dog food.

How are dog food and treat companies able to accomplish this? Tens of millions of dollars have been spent to produce a more palatable product to tantalize your pet. As the dog food and treat market has grown, so has the competition for new, novel, and highly desired products. Unfortunately, this competition has also spawned products that are less than nutritious and downright dangerous.

Is Your Dog Hungry, or Is It the Kibble Crack?

For a food scientist, the term "palatable" refers to the ability to encourage a dog's appetite and to prompt a dog to eat more than it needs. This definition doesn't include the concept of hunger. Both in the wild and in the food manufacturing plant, hunger is a negative and potentially dangerous physiological state. In the wild, if an animal does not develop an "appetite" or desire for food and energy prior to the onset of hunger, it may become weak or experience low blood-sugar levels that put that animal at a distinct disadvantage when it needs to seek out food. From an evolutionary perspective, then, appetite should naturally precede the hunger state. In this way, hunger is simply a biological protective mechanism. Unfortunately, this mechanism can be manipulated, and pet food manufacturers have done a remarkable job at it, creating in the process a nation of Chow Hounds.

If palatability is the ability to create an appetite, you can see how easily humans can override a dog's natural biological system. If we produce an extremely palatable food, a dog will pursue it regardless of its physiological needs. In other words, humans have the ability to make dogs eat more than they need and when they don't physiologically need or want more.

So what do dogs like? While this question is complex and controversial, we know that dogs, like many animals and humans, have evolved to prefer foods high in sugar, fat, and salt.

> **JUST THE DOGGONE FACTS**
>
> Dogs have about 1,700 taste buds, compared to over 9,000 in humans. It takes the average dog about a minute to consume one cup of dry dog food, while humans spend over eighty minutes per day eating and drinking.

The Terrible Trifecta: How Sugar, Fat, and Salt Make Your Dog Overeat

Sugar, fat, and salt present many problems for dogs. The primary concern is that sugar and fat contribute greatly to weight gain because they are higher in calories. However, even more dangerous is that when many animals eat foods rich in sugar, fat, or salt, they want to eat *more*, regardless of whether or not they should. In other words, sugar, fat, and salt increase a food's palatability to such an extent that most animals, including humans, eat more than they require—even when they're full.

Scientific studies confirm this statement. In a 1997 article published in the *American Journal of Physiology*, researchers studied two strains of rats and the impact of sugar and fat on their appetite and weight. The first group of rats was bred to become obesity-prone and would eat as much food as offered, while the second group did not typically overeat when offered a high-calorie diet.

In the study, researchers fed both strains of rats a high-fat diet. As expected, the obesity-prone rats engorged themselves while the obesity-resistant rats tended to eat only what they needed. Then researchers offered both groups of rats a diet that was high in fat *and* sugar. In this portion of the study, both groups of rats ate excessively. While this result was expected in the obesity-prone strain, researchers were surprised at the actions of the obesity-resistant strain. The conclusion was that the combination of high fat and high sugar levels in food overrides the body's normal regulatory systems to curtail appetite. Thus, even the rats bred to resist gaining weight became obese when offered sugar and fat. The same thing is happening to your dog.

While we don't fully understand the processes involved, we know that certain foods initiate release of a primary reward chemical in the brain called dopamine. In fact, the association between food and dopamine is so strong that many studies have compared the dopamine-release effects of food to drugs such as cocaine. Just as certain drugs elevate dopamine and cause forms of pleasure, increasing levels of sugar provide a similar response in the brain. In effect, high-sugar foods combined with high-fat foods act like a drug, causing your dog to want more food than it needs.

As far back as 1938, one of the twentieth century's most influential psychologists, Dr. B. F. Skinner, observed the dramatic impact that salted peanuts or potato chips had on his test animals when encouraging them to pursue additional rewards. He found that after the animals had stopped pursuing their normal food reward, usually a bland chow or pellet, they would perk up and seek these rewards again when he offered them a salty treat. Skinner didn't know that dopamine was behind these renewed efforts; he just knew the animals worked harder to get salty food rewards, despite being full or tired. Skinner's work was confirmed in the 1990s when Japanese researchers fed study dogs plain food and then food high in sugar and salt. The study food created such a response that the dogs stopped eating the plain study food altogether and would only eat the sugary and salty food.

 EYE ON THE SCIENCE

The Brain and Food Rewards

SOME OF THE MOST GROUNDBREAKING RESEARCH on the dopamine-food-reward feedback loop has occurred in the last decade. Neuroscientists have identified a particular region of the brain, the *nucleus accumbens*, which is highly involved in the food reward mechanism and is closely associated with dopamine. Moreover, the food reward system appears to involve additional areas of the brain, especially the *caudate nucleus*, a region that scientists believe is involved with human love and Obsessive-Compulsive Disorder. Because food reward involves complex brain chemistry and several regions of the brain, developing a safe and efficacious weight-loss or appetite-inhibiting drug for both pets and people has been challenging.

The fact that food components have the ability to change your dog's brain is most alarming. Just as we are witnessing a generation of humans who have developed the habit of overeating highly palatable foods, we are also seeing a generation of dogs conditioned to overeat. Super-palatable dog foods encourage our dogs to eat well beyond their needs. Many dog foods have become the equivalent of drugs to many of our pets, and we inadvertently continue to support their habit.

Love at First Bite

Do dog food companies add sugar, fat, and salt to their products? You bet they do. They're battling for a piece of the very lucrative pet food pie: In 2007, Americans spent more than $7 billion on dry dog food, $1.5 billion on wet food, and $2.2 billion on dog treats, for a total of $10.7 billion on dog food and goodies. If your dog appears to love a product, you're more likely to buy another bag or can. It's all about the first bite.

"First-bite preference" is an important term if you're in the business of designing dog food. Food palatability trials determine if a dog food will sell. Because dog food companies understand that their customer, the dog owner, is watching that first bite closely, they do everything to ensure their food is consumed rapidly and the dog appears to want more. Since our pet dogs typically aren't starving or even experiencing hunger, techniques that enhance palatability or the spontaneous consumption of a product are fair game. After all, that first bite *is* the game.

> " Just as we are witnessing a generation of humans who have developed the habit of overeating highly palatable foods, we are also seeing a generation of dogs conditioned to overeat. Super-palatable dog foods encourage our dogs to eat well beyond their needs. Many dog foods have become the equivalent of drugs to many of our pets, and we inadvertently continue to support their habit. "

Palatability

TO DETERMINE FIRST-BITE PREFERENCE, animal technicians offer a dog two identical bowls containing different foods at the same time. The technician records which bowl the dog eats from first. This is the first-bite preference that dog food manufacturers desperately need. The bowls are switched from left to right each day in the event that the dog has a preference for a particular side. Any remaining food is weighed and compared to the beginning weight. Most palatability studies are conducted during a five-day period. Some dog food companies perform additional at-home palatability studies with trained dog owners reporting their dog's feeding results to the researchers. The data is then compiled, and palatability scores are given for the foods. Unfortunately, it's the best-tasting food that wins, not necessarily the most nutritious one.

Why Dogs Like What They Like

In addition to the taste of the ingredients, factors such as kibble size and consistency, color, shape, and smell all contribute to whether a dog eats a given food. Just because something tastes good to humans does not mean that it will taste good to dogs. Certain breeds of dogs have shown preferences for specific food shapes, kibble size, and breaking point—the force required to crush and chew a kibble.

Another common observation is that puppies tend to prefer whatever food they were fed after being weaned. In fact, many owners of new puppies complain that their new puppy will only eat the food they received from the breeder. Research proves that puppies fed a limited number of flavors during the first four to six months of life are less likely to accept new flavors later on. The extent of this influence is determined by the palatability of the new foods offered. Most dog owners make this mistake: not feeding a variety of flavors during puppyhood.

Dogs fed an assortment of flavors are known to be neophilic. "Neophilia" is a term used to describe a person or animal that accepts new things and is excited by novelty. In reality, this is a good thing for omnivores; they seek out new tastes. The trouble starts when we fail to provide a variety of tastes for puppies. Over time, "diet monotony" or "flavor fatigue" develops, which leads dog owners to pursue more palatable foods over time. Because these flavor-deprived pups aren't used to new flavors contained in whole foods, they often prefer a series of ever-increasing fatty, sugary, and high-calorie diets during their lifetime. Owners do this because of their perception of their dog's first bite and the desire to make their dog as happy as possible. While we certainly have happy dogs in terms of providing super-palatable foods, we are creating very unhappy and unhealthy dogs in the long run. It simply doesn't make sense to start the cycle of a lifetime of pain, illness, and expensive medical treatments for the less than sixty seconds of pleasure your dog derives from consuming a cup of dog food.

Tweaking Taste Buds— From Protein Lovers to Sugar Junkies

How do dog food companies use this information on taste and smell to influence you and your dog's food choices? Packaging, social concerns, and kibble color are key influencers of the dog owner when choosing a dog food. For dogs, taste and smell are arguably the top two reasons they like or dislike a dry dog food. Therefore, dog food companies do everything in their power to influence that first bite, including adding ingredients a normal dog would never need.

In two studies conducted twenty years apart, in 1983 and 2003, researchers discovered a startling fact about dogs and their food choices. When dogs

> **❝ When dogs are given a choice to select their diets, they typically consume 25 percent to 30 percent of their calories from protein. ❞**

are given a choice to select their diets, they typically consume 25 percent to 30 percent of their calories from protein. These findings have been widely reported and used by the media, veterinarians, and pet food manufacturers.

What is not widely reported is that the study included experiments comparing the choice between a protein-free diet with and without added sucrose (sugar) and a protein-rich diet. When dogs were offered the choice of a diet with no protein and 6.4 percent sugar versus a protein-containing diet with 6.4 percent sugar, they chose the diet with protein. However, when the sugar content of the protein-free diet was increased to 25 percent, dogs more than doubled their preference for the protein-free diet. In fact, one-third of the dogs chose the food that contained no nutritive value other than sugar. It's easy to see why sugar can be used to sell food.

Dry dog food outsells canned dog food in the United States over four-to-one. While canned or moist dog food seems intuitively more appealing, at least to humans, dry dog food sells because of convenience. Think about it: a bag of dry dog food can be produced cheaply from a variety of food sources, and is easy to ship, store, and preserve. There are no messes or strong odors; it's easy and fast to serve and requires little thought. Simply pour some in a bowl and you're done. How's that for convenient?

One of the problems with dry dog food is that it bears little resemblance to anything natural. It really looks nothing like food. What meats, grains, vegetables, or fruits come in a half-inch cube, rectangle, star, or other cute shape? While this probably has no practical implication for puppies raised on dry food because that's all they've ever known (to them, dry kibble is food), it does factor into a dog owner's choice and overall palatability to the dog. As we've already learned, dogs have distinct preferences for kibble size, shape, and the amount of force required to chew. Dogs want their food to be as appealing as possible, after all.

People love brightly colored objects. But what about dogs? Do they care if their food is yellow and green and brown and star-shaped? Probably not. The fact is dogs don't even see the same colors humans do, so those red meaty chunks and green stars are lost on your dog. According to the latest research, dogs are most likely red-green color blind; they see blues and yellows really well, but greens and red may be misinterpreted as another hue. In general terms, your dog relies much more on its sense of smell in selecting food than the color of the kibble.

> ❝ People love brightly colored objects. But what about dogs? Do they care if their food is yellow and green and brown and star-shaped? Probably not. The fact is dogs don't even see the same colors humans do, so those red meaty chunks and green stars are lost on your dog. ❞

Despite this most obvious biological fact, food producers understand that humans buy dog food. Because humans rely heavily on visual cues to select foods, dog foods are made in the colors we find appealing. Some commonly used synthetic colors in dog food include:

Iron oxide

Coal tar derivatives known as Azo dyes

- Tartrazine (FD&C yellow no. 5)
- Sunset yellow (FD&C yellow no. 6)
- Allura red (FD&C red dye no. 40)

Non-Azo dyes

- Brilliant blue (FD&C blue no. 1)
- Indigotin (FD&C blue no. 2)

Artificial color(s)

No one knows for sure how safe or unsafe artificial colors may be. Most agencies, including the Food and Drug Administration (FDA), consider them safe. My advice is to avoid as many artificial colorings as possible. Chances are your dog won't know the difference.

Aside from the limited tweaks manufacturers can perform on the physical characteristics of dog food, the real prize lies with taste and smell. Modern food production science has provided manufacturers with almost limitless choices in how they can produce foods. In fact, most of the tastes and smells in today's processed human and dog foods are entirely synthetic. That's right, there's no need to add grape to a product when you can add methyl anthranilate (MA). What about meat? The Association of American Feed Control Officials (AAFCO) guidelines for dog food production allow a food to be called "beef-flavor" as long as the ingredients are sufficient to "impart a distinctive characteristic" to the food. Unfortunately, this means that a dog food can mislead consumers by being named "sirloin flavor" while actually containing no sirloin. All a dog food manufacturer must do is to include some beef product or by-product in their food, add a synthetic or natural flavor, and presto, "sirloin flavor" dog food is created. Food companies from McDonald's to Purina use flavoring agents to enhance the palatability of their foods. Taste buds are easy to fool.

The Nose Knows

In a benchmark study at Cornell University, researchers fed beagles a bland diet with odorless air blown across it alongside the same bland diet with meat odor blown over it. Initially, dogs preferred the bland food with meat odor 70 percent more than the odorless diet. By week three of the study, the preference dropped to 52 percent. Odor plays a significant role in first-bite preference of a food. The study also shows that dogs need more than an appealing smell to sustain their appetite for a given food, but aroma goes a long way.

Another part of the study that is rarely discussed is the impact that adding sugar or sucrose had on the dog's preference. In light of our recent understanding of the power of sugar in creating palatability, these findings from over thirty years ago have renewed relevance. The study beagles had their sense of smells temporarily disrupted using a nasal solution. When they couldn't smell, they didn't show a preference for one meat over another. However, when sugar was added to their diet, they demonstrated a preference for the sugary diet over the blander diet, regardless of whether they could smell. We now better understand why adding sugar plays a very important role in preference and palatability.

Another factor that is well-documented but poorly understood involves the tastes and smells a dog experiences in the womb and the impact this exposure has on flavor preferences. This phenomenon, pre-natal chemosensory learning, has been observed in many mammals, including humans, dogs, cats, sheep, rabbits, and mice. Studies as far back as the 1970s demonstrate that mammals prefer the tastes and smells to which they are exposed *in utero*. Thus, whatever a nursing mother eats influences the flavor preferences of her litter. Pet food companies know, "If we win the mother, we win the litter." Many pet food companies aggressively court breeders for this reason, something for dog owners to consider.

Read the Labels: Sugar and Fat

If you look closely at the ingredient labels of the top-selling dog foods, you'll begin to see a pattern. Because a dog food must be highly palatable and secure that coveted first-bite preference, dog foods, espe-cially dry kibbles, must pull out all the stops. Forget eating your veg-gies; today's dogs get mainly dessert at every meal (and between) because we dog lovers can't bear the thought that our dog doesn't instantly devour the food we provide. This psychology makes dog food production more challenging and leads producers to add ingredients, especially added fat, to meet this demand—often resulting in less healthy, but more palatable, foods. If you see either sugar or fat in the top ten ingredients, you'll know they are a major contributor to what you're feeding your dog—and that's not necessarily a good thing.

Is Sugar and Fat Lurking In Your Favorite Dog Food?	
Beneful Original Dry Dog Food	Animal fat: fifth ingredient Sugar: ninth ingredient
Iams ProActive Health™ Chunks	Chicken fat: fifth ingredient
Kibbles 'n Bits Original	Animal fat: fifth ingredient Corn syrup: sixth ingredient
Ol' Roy Dinner Rounds Dog Food	Corn syrup (a form of sugar): fifth ingredient Animal fat: eighth ingredient
Pedigree Adult Complete Nutrition for Dogs	Animal fat: fourth ingredient
Purina Dog Chow	Animal fat: third ingredient

Not surprisingly, canned dog foods typically have a much higher fat content than dry foods. Because high-fat diets are highly palatable to dogs, canned foods need not resort to adding sugar to their foods. To aid in concealing the actual fat content of canned foods, though, dog food manufacturers report fat content as-fed "crude fat." Basically they report how much fat is in the food diluted in added water. This gives a much lower value than the actual amount in the food.

Because water has no nutrients, an increase in the moisture content reduces the relative amount of fat, protein, or whichever nutrient you are measuring. Dry matter is whatever is left over after the water or moisture is removed. Evaluating a pet food on its "dry-matter basis" is the most meaningful way to assess its nutrient content. "Dry matter" is regulation-speak for "food."

Dry-matter basis relates to the way the body uses food. Imagine you're eating a moist piece of pie. Your body quickly absorbs the water;

the ingredients—nutrients, proteins, carbohydrates (sugars), and fats—remain for the body to use. The "moistness" of the pie doesn't make you fat; the ingredients in the pie add the pounds. To calculate the impact of the food's nutrients, we remove the water by using a dry-matter conversion.

The FDA advises pet owners to compare pet foods on a dry-matter basis as this is the only meaningful way to evaluate pet foods. What is puzzling is why the FDA doesn't make this process easier for the consumer and require pet food companies to list dry-matter values on the label.

Nightmare Math: Why Pet Food Labels Don't Compute

Imagine you have a cube of dried meat and a bowl of water. Analyzing the cube of meat, you find that it contains 25 percent protein and 20 percent fat. This is dry matter. Next, take that cube of meat, grind it up, and mix it with water. For this example, we'll say that the mixture is now 80 percent water and 20 percent meat. In food-label terms, this is the same as saying "80% maximum moisture." If you analyze this water/meat mixture, you find that the label says "crude protein content = 5.0%" and "crude fat content = 4.0%." Confusing, isn't it?

While Chapter 7 gives specific guidelines on what to feed your dog for weight loss, the chart that follows shows you how much the actual contents vary when you understand this fuzzy math. In fact, when you learn to calculate nutrients based on dry-matter basis, you'll notice that the fat content of most pet foods increases significantly. For weight loss, you should choose a food with a fat content as low as possible, generally 7 to 12 percent; less than 9 percent is ideal. For healthy, adult, indoor, spayed or neutered dogs, a fat content of 7 percent to 20 percent is recommended. More active dogs may require more fat in their diets.

EYE ON THE SCIENCE

Dry-Matter Calculation

TO CALCULATE DRY-MATTER NUTRIENT VALUES, follow this "simple" equation, which stumps many vets and vet technicians.

Dry Matter equals Nutrient percent as fed, divided by Reciprocal of the Moisture percent

If you look at a dog food label, you'll find something like this:

Guaranteed Analysis:

Protein 25%	Fiber 2%
Fat 12%	Moisture 10%

To calculate protein on a dry-matter basis (the actual amount of protein in the food) you need to first subtract the water:

100–10 (% moisture) = 90 (the reciprocal of Moisture)

This food is 90 percent dry matter. Most wet or canned foods contain about 78 percent moisture and only about 22 percent dry matter.

Next, take the percentage of protein from the label and divide it by the dry-matter percentage.

Dry-Matter-Basis Protein = 25 ÷ 90

Multiply that value by 100 to obtain a dry-matter-basis percentage of the nutrient.

Dry-Matter-Basis Protein = 25 ÷ 90 = 0.277 x 100 =

28 percent protein in the food on a dry-matter basis

Repeat the calculation for any nutrient.

Dry-Matter-Basis Fat = 12 ÷ (100–10) = 0.133 x 100 =

13.3 percent actual fat in the food when water is removed

Table 2.2. The Difference Between Fat on the Label and the Actual Fat Content

Type of Food	Name	Maximum Moisture Content (Percentage)	Minimum Crude Fat Content Reported on Label (%)	Actual Fat Content on Dry-Matter Basis (%)
Dry Food	Pedigree Adult Complete Nutrition for Dogs	12	10	11.4
Canned Food	Pedigree Butcher's Selects Premium Ground Entrée Filet Mignon Flavor	78	7	31.8
Dry Food	Iams ProActive Health™ Chunks	10	15	16.7
Canned Food	Iams Ground Savory Dinner with Meaty Beef & Rice	78	6	27.3
Dry Food	Purina ONE Small Bites Beef & Rice Formula	12	16	18.2
Canned Food	Purina ONE Wholesome Beef & Brown Rice Entrée	78	7	31.8
Dry Food	Hill's Science Diet Adult Small Bites Dry Dog Food	10	13	14.4
Canned Food	Hill's Science Diet Canine Beef & Chicken Entree	78	3	13.6
Dry Food	Nutro Max Beef Meal & Rice Dinner Dry Dog Food	10	16	17.8
Canned Food	Nutro Max Beef & Rice Dinner for Dogs	78	6.5	29.5
Dry Food	Beneful Adult Dog Food	14	10	11.6

Table 2.2 *(continued)*

Type of Food	Name	Maximum Moisture Content (Percentage)	Minimum Crude Fat Content Reported on Label (%)	Actual Fat Content on Dry-Matter Basis (%)
Canned Food	Beneful Prepared Meals Simmered Beef Entree with Carrots, Barley, Wild Rice & Spinach Dog Food Tubs	78	2	9.1
Dry Food	Newman's Own Organics Adult Dog Chicken Formula Dry Dog Food	10	12	13.3
Canned Food	Newman's Own Organics Adult Chicken Formula Canned Dog Food	78	6	27.3
Dry Food	Kibbles 'n Bits Beefy Bits Dry Dog Food	18	8	9.8
Canned Food	Kibbles 'n Bits Tender Cuts with Real Beef & Vegetables in Gravy	82	3	16.7

Fat isn't entirely bad. Dogs require fat in their diet not only for energy but also to supply essential fatty acids (EFAs) that their body cannot produce otherwise. The issue with these ingredient lists is that they most often represent *added processed fats*—fat in the form of grease, oil, or lard added to the mixture because there isn't much real meat in the food. These fake fats enhance texture and palatability and encourage your dog to eat more.

Think of it in these terms: 100 grams or 3.5 ounces of lean (1/8" trimmed) sirloin typically contains about 13 grams of fat and 20 grams of protein. That's a good amount of both fat and protein and one of the reasons dogs prefer beef protein. AAFCO requires a minimum 5.0 percent fat content in adult maintenance dog foods. Why add fat if the dog food is animal-based protein? Three reasons: (1) there isn't much meat in dog foods, and therefore not much naturally occurring fat; (2) to supply missing essential fatty acids (EFAs); and (3) to enhance palatability by improving flavor and texture.

Moist and semi-moist foods often have more added fat and sugar primarily because a sealed container resists spoilage better than exposed dry kibble. When canning technology was developed, manufacturers could suddenly formulate foods that would tempt even the most finicky dog.

Table 2.3. Sugar and Fat in Moist Dog Foods	
Purina's Moist & Meaty Chopped Burger Food	High-fructose corn syrup (a form of sugar): second ingredient Corn syrup (a form of sugar): seventh ingredient
Beneful® Healthy Harvest®	Animal fat: fourth ingredient Sugar: tenth ingredient
Bil-Jac Select Dog Food	Cane molasses (a form of sugar): seventh ingredient
Dad's Healthy Homestyle: Beef & Veggie Flavor Dog Food	High-fructose corn syrup: sixth ingredient
Kibble Select Complete: Premium Original with Beef/Chicken/Vegetable/Fruit & Cheese Dog Food	High-fructose corn syrup: fourth ingredient

The lesson here is to read closely the ingredient list of the food you're feeding your dog and avoid added sugar and fat whenever possible.

Rest assured, a select number of dog foods are produced with your dog's health and well-being, along with your convenience, in mind, and you can find in Chapter 7 my current top choices for weight-loss diets incorporating these foods. Unfortunately, as the stakes escalate in this multibillion-dollar industry, dog food companies become more clever and manipulative as they seek the first bite that translates into a sustained buy.

The Trouble with Treats

Have you ever watched what your dog does when she knows you're about to give her a treat? Most dogs stand on their rear legs, turn in circles, bark excitedly, or display extreme "happiness" if you even gesture toward a box of treats. I have patients that respond this way if they simply hear the word "treat." This classic Pavlovian conditioning comes from a very strong reward-stimulus: a sugar, fat, and salt goody. While many dog owners view this experience as positive, the fact is that this exaggerated response is abnormal and potentially destructive. What elicits joy for the dog is ultimately harmful and life-shortening. In reality, our dogs have become addicted to these sugary sweets as if they were habit-forming drugs (For a list of healthy treat alternatives, see chapter 8). The way for a company to win the war for dog-treat dollars is to produce a treat that dogs love, and the surest way—unfortunately—is to boost the amount of sugar, fat, and salt in the treats.

The Birth of the Dog Biscuit

In the mid-1800s, an entrepreneur by the name of James Spratt was about to revolutionize the dog food industry by creating an insatiable demand for a product no one knew they needed, and which would forever change how we interact with our dogs. Like many Americans in the mid-1800s, the Chicago native was determined to make a name for himself in the emerging world of business. As many young men had done a generation before, Spratt embarked in 1860 on a trans-Atlantic voyage to seek his fortune in Europe.

That same year, the Royal Society for the Prevention of Cruelty to Animals established the first Home for Lost and Starving Dogs just off Liverpool Road. Spratt was a dog lover. More important, he was ambitious.

As he disembarked from the ship in Liverpool, he saw packs of street dogs scavenging for discarded hardtack from docked ships. Hardtack is a simple cracker or biscuit, about three inches square, made of flour, water, vegetable fat, and salt. When freshly baked, hardtack is quite tasty. Because salt preserves hardtack well, the biscuits can resist spoilage. As it ages, hardtack becomes progressively harder, resulting in a staple foodstuff that sailors know as "tooth dullers" and "molar breakers."

When ships docked, the crew would often throw these despised biscuits into the dockside streets. Watching dogs scarf down discarded hardtack, Spratt had an entrepreneurial epiphany. He would produce and sell something better. But he wasn't a baker.

To begin his quest, Spratt devised a plan. To create his concept of a "dog biscuit," he enlisted the help of a packaging company popular with the English foxhound trade. Soon, Spratt's Patented Meat Fibrine Dog Cake was the seminal product of what would become the multibillion-dollar dog food industry. His recipe called for a mixture of blended wheat meals, vegetables, beetroot (sugar), and meat.

The source of meat used in Spratt's dog biscuits was a closely guarded secret. According to C. H. Lane in the 1902 book *Dog Shows and Doggy People,* even after Spratt had sold his business, until the time of his death in 1878, he kept in his hands the contract for his meat supplier.

Whatever the source of meat, Spratt had virtually overnight created demand for a product that was previously unnecessary. Pet dogs had historically been fed leftover food from human meals and left to forage on their own for additional food. Over the next 100 years, feeding a dog table foods or leftovers would become viewed almost as negatively as neglecting your own children. Overlooked was the fact that this shift may have been created in the name of profit.

Regardless of Spratt's motives, he returned to the United States to grow his dog food company. He was so successful that by 1895 he had to move his company to a new, larger building in Newark, New Jersey. Success breeds imitation. Enter F. H. Bennett.

In 1907 Bennett was struggling to sell his dry dog biscuits against the better-known Spratt's "dog cakes," which were available in several varieties. Bennett owned F. H. Bennett Biscuit Company—later Wheatsworth Bakery, which still operates today baking Wheatsworth Crackers. His bakery was in serious disrepair and barely functioning on antiquated equipment. During his first year, fire damaged his operations, delaying production for months. He needed a break.

While Bennett was interested in health and wanted to produce the most nutritious dog biscuits possible, he was competing against Spratt's giant company. In order to succeed, Bennett needed to do something different. Bennett didn't realize it at the time, but he made a move of marketing genius: instead of competing on the merits of his ingredients versus Spratt's, which were fairly similar, Bennett created differentiation based on shape. Dogs were probably unconcerned about the biscuit's shape of the biscuit, but dog owners took notice. Bennett made his biscuits in the shape of a bone. His "Malatoid Milk-Bones" were such a success that for the next fifteen years Bennett's Milk-Bone dominated the commercial dog food market in America.

During this time, American dog owners' feelings about their pets also began to evolve from viewing them as mere animals to their becoming companions. Spratt and Bennett were fortunate in that their newly created industry coincided with a period of national financial expansion and a positive change in society's perspective of dogs. It was a great time to be in the dog food business.

In 1931, the National Biscuit Company (Nabisco) purchased Milk-Bone from Bennett. Nabisco drew upon its large grocery store sales force to promote Milk-Bones initially as "a dog's dessert." They later changed their marketing to advertise the "breath-sweetening" properties of Milk-Bones.

This idea of "a dog's dessert" played right into the hearts of a changing public conscience. Dogs were becoming family members, and didn't we offer sweets and desserts to loved ones?

Dog treats today have come a long way from the original Milk-Bones, and the evolution hasn't always been positive. Bennett's Milk-Bones wouldn't stand a chance against today's dog biscuits. The treats lining grocery store shelves today are packed full of health-threatening levels of sugar, fat, and salt. If I had to place a bet, metaphorically, on spinach or dessert, my bet is on dessert. The $2.2 billion dog-treat market says I'm right.

The Lure of Sugar

In a 2001 study at Princeton University, researchers gave rats intermittent access to sugar water in addition to their normal food. The researchers found that when they discontinued the sugar water, the rats demonstrated behavioral and blood chemistry changes similar to those of withdrawal in drug-addicted rats. When the sugar solution was suddenly stopped, the rats would shake their heads, their forepaws trembled, their teeth chattered, and their bodies shook as if they were shaking off water. The study concluded that the rats had become sugar-dependent. Stopping the access to sugar led to anxiety and signs of withdrawal.

Another interesting but less-talked-about finding from the study involved the amount of sugar solution and food the rats ate. As the study progressed, rats ate more chow and consumed more sugar solution than when offered initially. Logic would dictate that the rats would eat less dry chow since they were receiving most of their calories from the glucose solution. The exact opposite occurred. On day one, rats ate 2.7 grams of chow during the first three hours. By day eight, that amount had skyrocketed to 10.5 grams—a 300 percent increase.

This study demonstrated that not only rats—but by extension humans, dogs, and many other mammals—become dependent on sugar, but that consuming more sugar leads to consuming more food in general.

Table 2.3. Are Your Doggie Treats Sugar Bombs in Disguise?			
Treat	Component(s) Added to Enhance Palatability	Reported Minimum Crude Fat Content on Label (%)	Actual Fat Content on Dry-Matter Basis (%)
Snausages	Corn syrup Snaw Somes! Beef and Cheese flavor: corn syrup: second ingredient sugar: third ingredient	1.5	2
Pup-Peroni Lean Beef Recipe	Sugar: third ingredient Salt: fifth ingredient	5	6.1
Meaty Bone dog biscuits	Animal fat: third ingredient Salt: sixth ingredient	5	5.7
Milk-Bone Traditional Small Dog Biscuits	Beef fat: sixth ingredient Salt: seventh ingredient	5	5.7
Milk-Bone Crunchy Mar-O-Snacks	Sugar: third ingredient Salt: seventh ingredient	7	8
Milk-Bone Bakery Bites Bacon Chip 'n Cheese Flavor	Sugar: third ingredient Beef fat: seventh ingredient Salt: tenth ingredient	4	4.6
Milk-Bone Natural Snacks	Dextrose (a form of sugar): third ingredient	2.5	2.8

Table 2.3 *(continued)*

Treat	Component(s) Added to Enhance Palatability	Reported Minimum Crude Fat Content on Label (%)	Actual Fat Content on Dry-Matter Basis (%)
Milk-Bone Jerky Strips	Sugar: fifth Ingredient	9	11.5
Greenies Smart Biscuit Double Green Chunk Dog Chew Treat	Poultry fat: fourth ingredient	5	5.6
Jerky Treats American Beef Dog Treat	Sugar: fourth ingredient Salt: seventh ingredient	8	10.5
Sergeant's Steak House Chippers Dog Treats	Poultry fat: second ingredient Corn syrup: eighth ingredient Dextrose: eleventh ingredient	10	12.5
Sergeant's Steak House Jerky Strips Dog Treats	Corn syrup: fourth ingredient Animal fat: eighth ingredient	10	13.9
Solid Gold Tiny Tots Jerky Dog Treats	Unrefined brown sugar: seventh ingredient Molasses: ninth ingredient Sea salt: tenth ingredient	5	7.1
Snausages Breakfast Bites Bacon and Egg Flavored Dog Treats	Sugar: sixth ingredient Corn syrup: ninth ingredient Salt: twelfth ingredient	4	5.7
Snausages Party Sack Dog Treat	Corn syrup: fourth ingredient Animal fat: eighth ingredient	7	10.1
Scooby Snacks Crunchy Dog Snacks for Medium-Large Dogs	Animal fat: third ingredient Salt: fifth ingredient	5	5.7

Table 2.3 *(continued)*

Treat	Component(s) Added to Enhance Palatability	Reported Minimum Crude Fat Content on Label (%)	Actual Fat Content on Dry-Matter Basis (%)
Purina T-Bonz Porterhouse Steak Flavor	Sugar: fifth ingredient	3	4.2
Authority Dental Wellness Dog Treats	High-fructose corn syrup (a form of sugar): fourth ingredient	2	2.9
Beefeaters Jerky Stix Dog Treats Bacon Flavor	Sugar: fourth ingredient Dextrose: fifth ingredient Salt: seventh ingredient	10	13.2
Old Mother Hubbard's Extra Tasty Dog Biscuits—Original Dog Biscuits	Chicken fat: third ingredient Molasses: fourth ingredient Sea salt: tenth ingredient	7	7.9
Exclusively Dog Vanilla Flavor Sandwich Creme Dog Cookies	Sugar, dextrose, salt: first three ingredients Corn syrup: sixth ingredient	16	17
Exclusively Dog Best Buddy Bones™ Beef & Liver Flavor Dog Treats	Sugar, vegetable fat, salt: second–fourth ingredients	14	15.2
Pedigree Jumbone Mini Snack Food for Small Dogs	Sugar: third ingredient	5	6.1
Eukanuba Healthy Extras Adult Maintenance Biscuits	Chicken fat: fourth ingredient	9	10.1
Bil-Jac Gooberlicious Dog Treats	High-fructose corn syrup: third ingredient	10	14.3

Now that you know how pet food manufacturers conspire against you and your dog, and how modern foods have turned many of our dogs into chow hounds, let's investigate in the next chapter what other dangers lurk in the murky world of pet food labels.

3

WHAT IS YOUR DOG EATING?
Deciphering Pet Food Labels

Here's a secret few veterinarians (or human doctors) will let you in on: most health professionals haven't the faintest clue how to interpret a food label. The situation is even more confusing when it comes to reading pet food and treat labels. The terminology used, the way in which they report nutrients, and even how they list ingredients are designed to confuse consumers and cloud the truth. If you aren't convinced, pick up your dog's food; try to decipher the label and attempt to explain to your neighbor, in plain English, exactly what's in the food. You're in for a challenge.

The situation is so bad that the notoriously conservative American Veterinary Medical Association (AVMA) issued a plea to the FDA on May 13, 2008, for help. In the request, the AVMA asks for sweeping changes in how pet food labels are prepared, including adding calorie statements on each food and treat. As of early 2010, no meaningful changes in pet food labels have occurred.

> ❝ Here's a secret few veterinarians (or human doctors) will let you in on: most health professionals haven't the faintest clue how to interpret a food label. ❞

To comprehend pet food labels, you'll need to wade through rules and regulations ranging from individual state guidelines to directives from many agencies with attractive acronyms, including:

- The U.S. Food and Drug Administration (FDA)
- The Department of Health and Human Services (HHS)
- The U.S. Department of Agriculture (USDA)
- The U.S. Federal Trade Commission (FTC)
- The Association of American Feed Control Officials (AAFCO)

To be sure, a lot of fingers are in the pet food regulation pie. While at first glance, a multitude of agencies overseeing pet food appears to be a good thing, and it generally is, making changes becomes nearly impossible as a result. To keep everyone happy and meet each agency's needs, plenty of concessions must be made. The end result is that something as simple as adding mandatory calorie statements to a bag of dog food or treats has—at the time of publication—yet to be implemented.

Who Regulates Dog Food and How Safe Is It?

At the federal level, the FDA and USDA are primarily in charge of ensuring the safety of pet foods purchased or exported from the United States. Few dog owners ever questioned the safety of dog foods until the massive pet food recall in 2007, when hundreds of dogs were poisoned by a toxic ingredient added to wheat gluten by manufacturers in China.

From that point on, pet owners began to scrutinize what they fed their dogs. Ultimately, ascertaining the safety of dog food is complicated. The FDA is in charge of ensuring that pet food intended for interstate sale is safe, and that pet food labels are truthful and accurate. Unfortunately, this inspection process may be more for show that they'd like you to know.

According to a *USA Today* report cited by California Senator Ellen Corbett in a failed bid to change pet food label requirements in 2008, the FDA inspects only approximately 1 percent of the imported food it regulates, down from a reported 8 percent in 1992. The report also revealed the FDA does not require countries exporting pet food to the United States to maintain safety systems equivalent to ours, even though the USDA has mandates for countries that wish to export meat and poultry to the United States. Finally, the report disclosed that from 2002 to 2007, food imports increased 50 percent while the number of FDA food-import inspectors dropped by approximately 20 percent.

Interestingly, pet foods don't require FDA approval before they are offered for sale. Of course, if a problem is found with a dog food after it is sold, the manufacturer faces severe consequences, which doesn't help your family if your dog suffers a complication or injury.

In order to justify the lack of pre-market inspection of pet foods, the government has established a standard for pet food ingredients called "Generally Recognized as Safe (GRAS) for their intended use." A dog food can be made from GRAS ingredients without any inspection. According to the FDA, "Many ingredients such as meat, poultry and grains are considered safe and do not require pre-market approval." Other food ingredients—such as minerals, vitamins, or other nutrients; flavorings and preservatives; or food-processing aids—are controlled by federal regulations or have been approved as food additives.

If you want to produce and market dog food, you simply need to buy some meat, bread, or vegetables; add any additives, colorings, flavorings, processing aids, and anything else you desire from the official lists; and take it for sale at your local pet supply store. I certainly don't recommend that you do this, but you could. As long as your food doesn't hurt a pet (at least that the government knows about), you won't be breaking any laws.

Even with this lax approach, the United States still has the safest food and drug supply in the world. The 2007 pet food recall and other recent human food and drug recalls simply show that we can do better.

As mentioned earlier, pet foods, unlike human foods, are also under the oversight of individual states. Another powerful group controls what is in your dog's food, too: the Association of American Feed Control Officials (AAFCO), arguably one of the most important animal food organizations in the world.

Table 3.1. Agencies Involved in Regulating Pet Food	
Association of American Feed Control Officials (AAFCO)	• Private organization that consists of government feed inspection officials; advised by pet industry and pet advocacy groups • Creates Model Bills used by most states to regulate pet foods • Works closely with FDA
U.S. Food and Drug Administration/ Center for Veterinary Medicine (FDA)	Regulates all pet foods involved in interstate commerce
State Feed Control Officials	Regulates all pet foods sold within the state
U.S. Department of Agriculture (USDA)	• Regulates imported pet foods • Inspects animal research facilities • Has a voluntary inspection system for pet food manufacturers
Federal Trade Commission (FTC)	Regulates print and electronic advertising of pet foods
National Research Council (NRC)	• Private organization created under the National Academy of Sciences (NAS) • Advises government agencies on scientific matters, including pet nutrition • Publishes "Nutrient Requirements of Dogs and Cats," a collection of current nutritional science findings and recommendations

The chief AAFCO lobbyist is the Pet Food Institute (PFI), a group of approximately thirty members who represent about 98 percent of all pet food production in the United States. Their stated purpose is to be an industry watchdog for any regulations that may negatively impact dog and cat food manufacturing as well as helping ensure that domestic pet foods are safe. If there is a challenge to anything related to pet foods, you can be sure the PFI will be the first to know and will act swiftly if the proposal goes against their members.

For example, in 2008, legislation was introduced into the California Senate that sought to change pet food labels. Legislators wanted manufacturers to include a toll-free number and website on their labels. In addition, the bill would require "processed pet food manufacturers and distributors" to include on their websites each ingredient used in their product with its country of origin, and where the pet food was processed, with the processor's name, location, and relevant contact information. Score one against pet owners.

Citing the expenses involved with passage of the bill, PFI worked closely with the California Manufacturers and Technology Association and Grocery Manufacturers Association and successfully defeated the bill.

The Influence of AAFCO and the FDA

AAFCO's primary function is to create examples of feed regulation that federal and state agencies may follow. AAFCO accomplishes this by publishing Model Bills, or boilerplate standards of animal food guidelines and codes that different jurisdictions can adopt.

In addition to Model Bills, AAFCO publishes recommended regulations to support the Model Bills, a list of definitions of ingredients used in animal feeds, and other tips for supervising animal food at the regulatory level. States can use the Bills as is; thirty-eight states, as of late 2009, do just that. Because the majority of states use some, if not all, AAFCO guidelines in their animal feed regulatory acts, AAFCO guidelines have nationwide influence.

AAFCO enters into the pet food label game by establishing levels of nutrients that the food must contain, the requirements for adequacy of foods for different life stages, and feeding directions. From there it gets progressively more complicated, despite both agencies' desire to make it easier for dog owners to understand what they're feeding. Call it a bureaucratic bog if you'd like; the labels are still difficult to decipher.

The FDA assists AAFCO with many scientific and technical issues related to pet nutrition. This close collaboration is especially important when it comes to AAFCO's ingredient definition procedure. These two agencies work together to ensure proposed new ingredients for use in pet foods are proven to be as safe as possible. If AAFCO approves a dog food ingredient, then it is basically acceptable to the FDA.

What Is "Complete and Balanced" Dog Food?

When you see the words "complete and balanced" on your dog food, that's AAFCO at work. There are three standards by which AAFCO will recognize a dog food as "complete and balanced," "perfect," or "100% nutritious."

1 The dog food contains the proper amount of nutrients determined by AAFCO for all life stages: gestation/lactation, growth, and adult maintenance.

2 The manufacturer proves the "nutritional adequacy" of a dog food by completing an AAFCO-recognized feeding trial.

3 If a new dog food is a member of a product "family" with a similar combination of ingredients to an existing AAFCO-approved food, the new formulation may automatically be eligible for the "complete and balanced" designation without any testing or analysis.

Meeting AAFCO Standards Is Voluntary

Meeting AAFCO standards is voluntary for the pet food manufacturer. In recent times, some dog food companies have opted not to seek AAFCO approval, citing the inadequacies and political nature of the organization. In truth, there are good and bad foods that are AAFCO-approved, and there may be just as many good and bad foods that are not AAFCO-approved. Consumers ultimately decide what matters most: the brand, the ingredients, or AAFCO. All the AAFCO approval tells you is that, through a variety of means (some more legitimate than others), the food has the basic nutrition your dog needs. Whether or not these nutrients are in the ideal amounts or even if they are digestible is not guaranteed by the simple words, "meets AAFCO standards."

A Confusing "Family"

When a pet food is grouped as part of a family of products, a pet food company can sell a dog food without doing much research on it. If a dog food manufacturer can prove that its new food is in an approved family and is similar enough to a "lead" product, the new food bypasses most testing. Paying lawyers and scientists to write papers about why a new food is in a "family" is far less expensive than conducting food analysis or feeding trials.

AAFCO regulations also allow manufacturers to boost levels of other ingredients in the family as long as they stay within the maximum and minimum levels. Unfortunately, *there is no maximum for fat content*. Once a lead product is established, the manufacturer can go back and add as much fat to the product as they wish, thus enhancing palatability and the appeal to your dog of those high fat and sugary foods they go nuts for—literally. Dog food producers can essentially use the skeleton formula of a previously approved lead product and dress it up with fat, carbohydrates, and protein without performing any additional feeding trials. In this way, companies can react to the time crunch of the market and quickly produce new versions of a dog food to meet consumer demands without the time and expense of additional feeding trials. There is a very good possibility that the exact food you're feeding your dog today was never fed to dogs in tests to see if it was healthy. If this much wiggle room exists in introducing a product to market, you can imagine how loosely controlled other attributes of dog food are.

> **There is a very good possibility that the exact food you're feeding your dog today was never fed to dogs in tests to see if it was healthy.**

Naming and Branding

AAFCO strictly regulates the ways in which dog foods are named and branded. The *2009 AAFCO Official Guide* contains 30 pages of rules regarding the labeling of animal food, and the *AAFCO Pet Food and Specialty Guide* devotes its entire 139 pages to help explain those regulations. The codes detail dog food packaging: where the type will be on the package; how large or small the words will be; what words may or may not be used; and the colors, fonts, and other fine points of design. All of these rules are an effort to keep dog food companies honest. Savvy marketing experts often bend and twist the rules designed to protect the public. Each year AAFCO tries to counter these marketing strategies by adding to the already voluminous regulations. Consider this troubling fact: AAFCO's 169 pages devoted to pet food labels dwarfs the 15 pages used to describe the nutrient profiles and their substantiation. In other words, the marketing attacks that influence your purchase far outweigh the nutritional concerns. In a perfect world, the regulatory debate wouldn't be about what a dog food is named but rather what it contains.

With all due respect to their authors, people interested in dog food ingredients and packaging must dig deeply through two hard-to-understand books to figure out the meanings of terms such as "meat by-products," "beef flavored," "organic," and "natural." All of this complexity and confusion is not entirely AAFCO's fault. As quickly as AAFCO officials can define and place limitations on a term, dog food marketers come up with another clever descriptor. It's a classic case of catch-me-if-you-can, with the power of the marketers always ready to answer the regulators.

Caveat Emptor: What's Really in a Name?

AAFCO labeling requirements provide definitions for words used to name or describe dog food—another foray into the murky waters of codes.

"100%" or "All"

Seeing "100%" or "All" on a label means the food is completely made up of that ingredient. It can contain no other ingredients, except water. An example would be a dog food claiming to be "100% Venison Dog Food." That dog food may only contain venison and sufficient water for packing. According to AAFCO rules, "Beef Dog Food" isn't required to be 100 percent beef unless it contains "100%" or "All" on the package.

The 95% Rule

Dog food companies aren't dumb: To get around the cost-prohibitive 100% Rule, they began employing clever word play. Dog food companies began naming their food "Beef Dog Food" when it actually contained only a small amount of beef. To prevent this, AAFCO created the "95% rule," which basically states that the ingredient(s) derived from animals, poultry, or fish must constitute at least 95 percent of the total weight of the product. Water sufficient for processing may be excluded when calculating the percentage; however, the ingredient(s) shall constitute at least 70 percent of the total product weight.

The first important fact about this rule is that it only deals with meat, poultry, or fish. Vegetables would not be covered under this rule.

While the rule seems to imply that the food contains "95%" of an ingredient, it doesn't exactly require that. If water is added, you remove the moisture, and the ingredient must then constitute at least 70 percent of the remaining total weight. A dog food meeting these requirements of at least 95 percent of the total weight or at least 70 percent of the total weight of beef when any added water is removed may be called "Dr. Ernie's Yummy Beef Dog Food."

In the *Pet Food Specialty Guide*, an important explanation appears regarding names and ingredients involved in the 95% Rule: feed officials should verify that the ingredient name used in the dog food or treat name is the same as the ingredient name used in the ingredient list. For example, a dog food can't be called "Beef Dog Food" if its main ingredient is beef by-product.

The 25% Rule

Dog food companies realized that adhering to the 95% Rule was expensive. They looked for ways to name their food "beef" or "chicken" while adding as little of these expensive ingredients as possible. Enter the "Entrée Rule."

The "Entrée" or 25% Rule states that if a dog food is called "dinner," "platter," "entrée," "formula," or "recipe," the main ingredient must equal 25% of the formulation not counting water sufficient for processing. For example, "Healthy Valley Beef Recipe Dog Food" must contain at least 25 percent beef. Strangely, a food adhering to the 25% rule doesn't actually have to contain 25% of a product. If two or more ingredients are listed, for example, "Healthy Valley Rice and Beef Dinner," both ingredients must add up to 25% with a minimum 3 percent for a listed ingredient. In reality, this food may contain as little as 3% beef and 22% rice to meet AAFCO label requirements. When it comes to the "Entrée Rule," one plus one is less than you'd think (at least in terms of beef).

If a dog food is named "Chicken and Beef Formula Dog Food," it's even more misleading. At first glance this name sounds very similar to "Chicken and Beef Dog Food." Most dog owners would rightly believe this was a dog food made up of mainly chicken and beef. They'd be wrong.

"Chicken and Beef Dog Food" must add up to 95 percent chicken and beef. Because of AAFCO regulations, "Chicken and Beef Formula Dog Food" may contain only 22 percent chicken and only 3 percent beef. Where's the beef in that? Must've gotten lost in the "Formula."

So whenever you see these terms on a dog food label, be aware that what looks like "beef" may contain very little meat. Marketing trumps pet nutrition once again, as approved under the AAFCO regulations.

The "With" Rule

As time marched forward, dog food manufacturers complained that 25 percent meat was too expensive. They still wanted to give dog owners the impression that their foods were "meaty" or contained lots of chicken and other nutritious ingredients; they just didn't want to include them. That cost too much.

Once again, AAFCO came to the rescue with Regulation PF(3)—the "With" or "3% Rule."

The "With Rule" allows a dog food to be named after a relatively minor ingredient, one constituting as little as 3 percent of the total product weight, after any water has been removed. Dog owners need to be aware of this rule because it is difficult to tell the difference between a truly meaty food such as "Dr. Ernie's Beef Dog Food" and one with relatively little meat "Dr. Ernie's Wholesome Dog Food with Beef."

Let's look at another example. "Dr. Ernie's Mediterranean Style Medley with Salmon and Rice" sounds healthy enough. The label displays a pink salmon steak perched upon a bed of steaming rice surrounded by colorful vegetables. I'm getting hungry just thinking about it! But upon closer inspection, this gourmet dog food lists salmon as its fourth ingredient, after three carbohydrates, and rice fifth. Because "with Salmon and Rice" is used, this food must contain only 3 percent salmon and 3 percent rice. "Made with Real Beef" and "Contains Real Chicken" are also often found on dog food labels and are examples of the "3% Rule." As good as a food may sound, if "with" appears in the name, you can bet your dog's nutrition is getting short-changed. By no more than 3 percent, that is.

As you begin to study dog food names and labels, you'll find that almost none meet the 100 or 95 percent rules, some adhere to the 25 and 3 percent rule and the majority follows my favorite rule, the "Flavor Rule."

My Favorite: The "Flavor Rule"

After some time, even adding 3 percent of an ingredient such as beef or chicken became cost prohibitive. Shrewd marketing experts contemplated that dog owners would believe "Beef Flavor" was the same as "Beef Dog Food." They were right. Adding a flavor is a lot cheaper than adding the actual ingredient.

AAFCO Pet Food Regulation PF3(d) allows pet food companies to use the word "flavor" in the following circumstances. A flavor designation may be used anywhere in the product name or on the package as long as the food or treat can substantiate it. The rule allows dog food makers to claim "beef flavor" without adding any beef.

Let's examine a new dog food, "Farmer George's Home Style Beef Flavor Dog Food." When you pick up the bag you see a kindly old farmer whom we presume is "George" patting his trusty (and exceptionally healthy) Labrador retriever on a warm and inviting front porch. Anyone would assume the dog food in the bag was made with beef. Good old, real American stick-to-your-ribs beef. Heck, Farmer George may have made the food himself.

According to the "Flavor Rule," Farmer's George's food isn't required to contain beef. As long as the list of ingredients, that tiny box on the side of the bag with all those confusing names, states where the "beef flavor" originates, all is well in AAFCO-regulation land. Farmer George doesn't have to add expensive beef to his food; he can add much cheaper "animal digest (source of beef flavor)," and plainly says so on his ingredient list. Worse, the animal digest itself doesn't even have to contain any beef as long as it imparts a beef flavor. (And just what is "digest" anyway?)

Claiming Calories

Dog foods are not required to contain a calorie statement. You read that right; putting the number of calories in a cup or can of dog food is voluntary. The only exception to this rule is if the dog food claims it is "light," "low calorie," or "reduced calorie."

AAFCO seems to be opposed to pet food labels listing their calories. In addition to not requiring calorie content on pet foods, they've also largely ignored the pleas request of consumer groups and the American Veterinary Medical Association. Further, even if a pet food company does include calories, the presentation is virtually impossible for consumers to understand.

The regulation that causes endless confusion among pet owners and veterinarians is AAFCO PF9(a)(2). It requires calories to be expressed "as is" and in terms of kilocalories per kilogram of food (kcal/kg), not calories in a cup or can.

This approach has led to the practice of some "diet" dog foods listing their calories in a virtually impossible-to-calculate "kilocalories per kilogram of product." For example, a bag of dry dog food contains, according to the label, "3024 kcal/kg of metabolizable energy (ME) on an as fed basis (calculated)." How do you determine how many calories are in a cup? By doing a lot of measuring and calculating. You start by weighing a cup of the food, then you calculate how many cups are in a kilogram of the food, and finally you determine how many calories are in a cup. The pet food companies know that no one's going to go to all that trouble. The result is that "Lite Dog Food" you're feeding may not be so light in calories after all. You can almost bet that if a "low calorie" diet food expresses its calories as "kcal/kg of metabolizable energy (ME) on an as fed basis," it's not really low in calories.

Calorie Word Games

Almost ten pages of rules in the *Pet Food Guide* deal with calorie terms alone. Some rules work; others merely confuse.

"**Light.**" Regulation PF10(a)(1)A outlines the use of the terms "light," "lite," "low calorie," and similar words or terms. As you may guess, the approved usage is challenging to decipher:

PF10(a)(1)(A)

Contain no more than 3100 kcal ME/kg for products containing less than 20% moisture, no more than 2500 kcal ME/kg for products containing 20% or more but less than 65% moisture, and no more than 900 kcal ME/kg for products containing 65% or more moisture.

If that regulation confuses you, you're not alone. This rule defines the number of calories that "low calorie" dog foods may contain. ME stands for "metabolizable energy" and is the number of calories (kcal) in each kilogram (kg) of food. Basically this is the number of calories in just under thirty-six ounces of food. The rule also makes adjustments for the food's moisture or water content. Since water has no calories, the actual food must contain fewer calories when analyzed "as fed" in water, because the water is part of the food's total weight. Thus, an ounce of dry food would appear to have more calories than an ounce of canned food because there is more food in the dry product. However, if you took the water out of the canned food and compared the food left over, you would be better able to compare the two foods, as discussed earlier in Chapter 2 regarding "dry-matter basis." No wonder your dog doesn't lose any weight eating "lite" dog food.

"Less" or "Reduced Calorie." What about claims that a dog food has "reduced calories"? Reduced from what? Fortunately a rule forbids a company from simply writing on the label "Super Diet Dog Food is now lower in calories!" Instead, the company can state, "Super Diet Dog Food now with 10% less calories than Original Formula" or "Super Diet Dog Food is 10% Lower in Calories Than Fido Formula One."

Unfortunately, this regulation does not require the terms "less calories" or "reduced calories" to adhere to the (somewhat pathetic) "light" or "low calorie" guidelines. In other words, a dog food can boldly proclaim "reduced calories" or "less calories" for a dog food that has twice the number of calories a dog needs, further confusing consumers and leading to overweight dogs.

"Lean" and "Low Fat." The regulation also addresses "lean," "low fat," and other similar words and terms. This should be easy, but while the rule defines "low fat," it doesn't go far enough.

The AAFCO Nutrient Profiles require a minimum of 5 percent crude fat for adult maintenance dog food. This amount of fat is needed in a diet to maintain weight and health in adult dogs. The regulation allows a low-fat dog food to contain up to almost double that amount or 9 percent for dry foods. Wet foods can contain no more than 4 percent crude fat. But when you adjust for moisture, that equals 18 percent fat on a dry-matter-basis. Even more interesting, AAFCO guidelines recommend only 8 percent fat be in a dog food for pregnant or lactating females or growing puppies. "Low fat" diets can have more fat than is recommended for growth.

Fat is an important part of a healthy dog's diet. My only concern is that the terms "lean" and "low fat" as currently defined may confuse dog owners. Dog food companies claim that it's challenging to formulate a food with low fat content, and they may be right. When you hear that argument, keep in mind that the government defines "lean beef" as containing about 10 percent fat. I don't know many dogs that would turn down a "lean" T-bone steak as defined by the USDA.

"Less fat" or "Reduced fat." The *AAFCO Pet Food Guide* defines how dog food companies may use the terms "less fat" and "reduced fat" on their labels. This is a rewrite of the "less" or "reduced calories" rule. It's only used to compare to a previous formulation of another food. There are ample opportunities to exploit this rule to make a not-so-weight-loss-friendly food appear more so. Buyer beware.

Beware of Low-Calorie Imposters: "Weight Management" Foods

Because consumer interest and demand in low-calorie and low-fat pet foods have escalated over the past few years, dog food companies want in on the action. Trouble is, they want in quickly and cheaply. In such a case, the "pet food family" and label regulations really come into play. Say you're a dog food maker and your latest sales numbers are down. Your data indicates that you're losing sales to a competitor's low-calorie offering. You don't have a comparable product. "No problem," says the marketing department. "Just create a family product with the same basic nutrient profile and leave the rest to us."

A few months later, after conducting the chemical analysis and paperwork, you've just launched a "New and Improved Weight Management Dog Food." Your company hires an advertising agency to promote your new food alongside thin, healthy, vivacious dogs and people with the tagline, "Manage Your Dog's Healthy Life with New Weight Management Diet." Dog owners are captivated by the television ads and flashy packaging, and your sales figures soar. Problem solved, profit made, and barely a dime spent on product research and development.

Dog companies have twisted terms such as "weight management" and "weight control" into meaning "low calorie" or "reduced calorie."

To the average consumer, "Low Calorie Dog Food" and "Weight Control Dog Food" both sound like diet food for dogs. One may be; the other most likely isn't.

Hopefully AAFCO will enact regulations on these new diet imposters. Even so, shrewd marketing departments probably already have ready and waiting the next round of word games designed to confuse dog owners. As concerned dog owners, the best you can do is write AAFCO, the AVMA, and your elected officials and tell them you're tired of the pet food label lies. It's time we get easy-to-understand labels and calorie counts that we can use on the foods and treats we give our pets.

How Natural Is "Natural"?

In marketing terminology, "natural" is used to describe something as "wholesome," "good," and, in food, "nutritious." Dog owners have been demanding increased "natural" products, and the dog food companies have delivered. But what exactly have they delivered? If you think you've been feeding your dog food made of whole, unprocessed, or unaltered ingredients, you're mistaken.

AAFCO defines the feed term "natural" in Section IV (B) of the *Pet Food Guide*.

> A feed or ingredient derived solely from plant, animal or mined sources
> . . .

So far, that covers about everything in the known universe. But the regulation goes on,

> . . . either in its unprocessed state or having been subject to physical processing, heat processing, rendering, purification, extraction, hydrolysis, enzymolysis or fermentation, but not having been produced by or subject to a chemically synthetic process and not containing any additives or processing aids that are chemically synthetic except in amounts as may occur unavoidably in good manufacturing practices.

If "natural" is anything "from plant, animal or mined sources," where's the problem? The problem is that modern dog food is made up more of additives and ingredients than of whole foods. Meat is "natural" and contains a variety of minerals and vitamins; the same goes for vegetables, grains, salt, and so on. Didn't dogs thrive for tens of thousands of years without the addition of synthetic or processed ingredients? Doesn't "real food" contain the proper nutrient levels for dogs? What this regulation actually provides is a way for pet food manufacturers to make a very unnatural finished product resemble a natural one, at least in name. If AAFCO really wanted to improve dog food, it would require that "natural" meant, well, natural.

> In these cases, the guidelines indicate the term "natural" may be used on the label, provided that the claim is qualified with a disclaimer statement to disclose that synthetic nutrients have been added to the product.

AAFCO is thus requiring dog food makers to state on the bag that it's not really "natural" but an amalgam of synthetic chemicals parading around as "natural." But consider the following example: "Granny's Country Kitchen Dog Treats with Natural Cheese Flavor." Sounds yummy—and healthy. Can't you just imagine Granny in her kitchen out in the country cooking up a plate of healthy treats for her dogs? Grannies typically use only fresh ingredients, and this granny even added natural cheese. What could be better, or more natural and wholesome for your dogs?

But all is not as it seems in Granny's kitchen. There is very little "natural" or healthy in her treats.

> Example 2: The term "natural" may also be used to describe a specific ingredient provided that the term refers only to that ingredient and not the product as a whole.

You can produce an entirely synthetic food, add a "natural" flavoring (it doesn't have to be a piece of actual cheese), and use the word "natural" in the name to make it appear healthier or more wholesome or whatever the consumer perceives it is. The example of the above treat is taken straight from the *AAFCO Pet Food Guide*. The only change was the name of the treat (from "Manufacturer") and from "cat" to "dog." Other examples in the *Pet Food Guide* provide additional ideas for using the term "natural" in pet foods. All is not as it seems in the "natural" world of dog foods.

"Organic" Is Good, Right?

According to the Organic Trade Association, Americans spent approximately $24.6 billion on organic food and nonfood products in 2008. A total of $22.9 billion (3.5 percent of money spent on all foods) was spent on organic foods, including pet foods. What are we paying for?

As of 2010, there are still no standards for organic pet foods. The National Organic Standards Board (NOSB) recommended in October 2004 that a Task Force be formed to develop labeling standards for organic pet food. This Task Force was formed in May 2005 and has been working on guidelines for organic pet foods ever since. The twelve-member Task Force is currently chaired by the vice president of the Pet Food Institute (PFI) and has only one feed control official. The other officer, the secretary, works for a company specializing in assisting companies to successfully obtain USDA National Organic Program (NOP) Organic Certification. The rest of the Task Force is made up of pet food consultants and pet food company representatives. The only veterinarian involved is a pet nutrition consultant. Draw your own conclusions. While the USDA isn't required to take the NOSB's recommendations from the pet-food company-heavy Task Force, it probably will.

Because of this confusion, you haven't seen a lot of the word "organic" in pet foods. But thanks to AAFCO, that situation may change soon. While the *AAFCO Pet Food Guide* points out that dog food companies should refrain from using the word "organic" relative to its foods, AAFCO offers a clever alternative: name the company "organic."

> The USDA does not regulate company names. However the USDA has stated they will monitor the use of the term "organic" in company names, and work with the Federal Trade Commission to take action against the misuse of the term.

There you have it: according to AAFCO, it's okay to name your company "organic." I completely disagree with this tactic. In human foods, for a food to be certified "organic," at least 95 percent of the ingredients must be organically produced. For dog foods labeled "organic" today, be very skeptical. We can only hope that one day soon dog foods will have meaningful definitions for "organic." This is a game with billions of dollars at stake. If a company can produce an "organic" product at a low price, it will sell. The problem is that it's extremely difficult, if not impossible, to produce truly organic food cheaply. If you find organic food at a price close to a similar food product produced nonorganically, you may not be getting what you think you are.

Can I Eat It? "Human Grade" and "Human Quality"

Dog food companies have recently been pushing the label war to new heights. The terms "human grade," "fit for human consumption," and "human quality" have begun appearing on dog food labels. For example, a dog food company might claim it uses "human grade chicken in its food." This approach is misleading because the terms are meant to imply that the entire product meets USDA and FDA standards for human edible foods. If you add a "human grade" ingredient to an inedible one, the entire product is considered inedible by the FDA.

This matter drew national headlines in 2007 when Ohio's Department of Agriculture prevented the Honest Kitchen from selling its food on the grounds that its food label was misleading. The Honest Kitchen claimed on its label to use "human-grade" ingredients, a term that has no strict legal definition. The Department of Agriculture argued that consumers would be misled into believing the pet food was made to the same high standards as human foods. The Honest Kitchen won on the basis of free speech and continues to use the term today. However, AAFCO updated its regulations in February 2008 to prohibit the use of these terms due to the potential confusion. Dog food companies still use the terms, usually in marketing materials and on their websites. "Our pet food uses human grade and fit for human consumption ingredients such as natural chicken and organic grains."

Because "human grade" has no legal definition, it is hard to interpret exactly what a dog food manufacturer has in mind when using it. Is it really an ingredient intended for humans, or just clever marketing? I am certainly supportive of using the highest-quality ingredients in dog foods; I'm also interested in truth in advertising. If you see these terms on the label, I recommend contacting the company to determine the exact ingredients it is using. Perhaps the USDA, FDA, and AAFCO can reach some clear consensus on the definition and use of these terms to better inform dog lovers.

Interpreting Ingredients

What most dog owners really want to know is what is in their pet's food. Unfortunately, the number of flavorings, colorings, and preservatives has skyrocketed. To make things more confusing, dog food manufacturers, in an effort to control costs, have been forced to find cheaper nutrient sources, rendering a dog food ingredient list looking more like a high school chemistry experiment.

Bewildering By-Products

Perhaps the most controversial ingredient is the by-product. Many pet advocacy groups and pet food companies denounce by-products as unhealthy, unnecessary, and dangerous. Some dog foods claim to contain "no by-products" and then list "poultry by-products" on the label.

By-products can be good and bad, healthy and unhealthy. To say all by-products are bad is misleading; to say they're all good is equally inaccurate. In fact, there's a great possibility you eat by-products every day. Flour, meals, glutens, grits, and oils are all considered plant by-products. Anything made from a part of a food source is technically a "by-product." What we refer to as "meat by-products" are actually considered delicacies in many countries. For example, organ meats such as liver, heart, and stomach are favored in many Asian countries. In the wild, wolves eat these fat- and protein-rich tissues first. And don't forget your beloved hot dog; a mash-up of some of the most questionable animal by-products coated in mustard and chili.

Most meat by-products are made by a process known as "rendering." Rendering is a cooking process that is essentially the same as boiling chicken to remove the fat. In the commercial setting, imagine huge rendering vats or pots into which meat is placed (and sometimes bones). The contents of the vat are boiled, and the fat is drained off the remaining soup. This fat may be used as lard for cooking or animal fat (often referred to as "tallow") added as an ingredient to other food. Any meat chunks, bones, or heavy particles are separated, often many times, from the leftover liquid. Once the boiling and separation of fat are complete, the remaining watery solution is dehydrated or dried. The leftover solid portion is then ground into a powdery "meal" that is rich in protein and contains no fat.

Poultry meal produced in this manner may contain every part of the chicken except the head, feet, intestines, or feathers. Meat meal (may be called beef meal, lamb meal, or after whatever animal is used to make the meal) is rendered in the same manner and is made of everything in the cow, sheep, or pig except any added blood, hair, hoof, horn, hide trimmings, manure, stomach, or rumen (stomach of cow or sheep). Fish meal may contain the entire fish, scales, bones—everything.

Rendering meats is advantageous in that little animal waste is produced and any waste is used as pet food ingredients. From an environmental standpoint, any production method that creates little waste is a good thing. From a nutritional standpoint, it's not ideal but acceptable.

A 1998 *Journal of Nutrition* study conducted at the University of Illinois examined the issue of using rendered animal by-products in dog food. The study concluded that beef and poultry by-products are good sources of highly digestible nutrients for dogs. The problem they found with animal by-products was that digestibility fluctuated greatly based on particular food production techniques, mixtures, and rendering processes. In general, beef by-products had higher digestibility than poultry by-products.

Knowing and trusting your dog food company is important. Some companies dump everything allowable into their foods, while others select only the healthiest by-products. Both appear identical on the ingredient list. Perhaps the biggest problem with many dog foods isn't the fact that they contain by-products, but that they aren't ideally formulated for optimal health.

The table that follows contains some of the more common AAFCO meat, poultry, and fish sources:

Table 3.2. Common AAFCO Dog Food Ingredients—Protein Source

Ingredient	AAFCO Definition	Interpretation
Meat		
*9.3 Meat By-Products (Proposed 1973, Adopted 1974, Amended 1978) IFN 5-00-395 Animal meat by-products fresh	The non-rendered, clean parts, other than meat, derived from slaughtered mammals. It includes, but is not limited to, lungs, spleen, kidneys, brain, livers, blood, bone, partially defatted low temperature fatty tissue, and stomachs and intestines freed of their contents. It does not include hair, horns, teeth and hoofs. It shall be suitable for use in animal food. If it bears the name descriptive of its kind, it must correspond thereto.	• Everything else except hair, horns, teeth, and hoofs. The phrase "is not limited to" ensures this. • The intestinal tract must be emptied before using the stomach and the small and large intestines. • If it is labeled "poultry by-products," it must come from chickens. • Good dog food may contain nutritious by-products while lower-quality dog food may contain less than nutritious by-products.
9.7 Animal liver (Adopted 1954, Amended 2006) IFN 5-00-389 Animal livers meal	If it bears a name descriptive of its kind, it must correspond thereto. Meal is obtained by drying and grinding liver from slaughtered animals.	• Liver tissue from specified animal. • Healthy by-product that is specifically included on ingredient list when used.
9.40 Meat Meal (Proposed 1971, Adopted 1972, Amended 1985, Adopted 1993) IFN 5-00-385	The rendered product from mammal tissues, exclusive of any added blood, hair, hoof, horn, hide trimmings, manure, stomach and rumen contents except in such amounts as may occur unavoidably in good processing practices. It shall not contain added extraneous materials not provided for by this definition. The Calcium (Ca) level shall not exceed the actual level of Phosphorous (P) by more than 2.2 times. It shall	• Rendering is a process that converts waste animal tissue into a usable food ingredient. • Any tissue other than blood, hair, hoof, horn, hide trimmings, manure, stomach, and rumen contents may be used. • Used to maximize utilization of animal carcass, leaving little waste. • Provides protein, calcium, and phosphorous and other nutrients.

Table 3.2. Meat *(continued)*

9.40 Meat Meal *(continued)*	not contain more than 12% pepsin indigestible residue and not more than 9% of the crude protein in the product shall be pepsin indigestible. The label shall include guarantees for minimum crude protein, minimum crude fat, maximum crude fiber, minimum Phosphorous (P) and minimum and maximum Calcium (Ca). If the product bears a name descriptive of its kind, composition or origin, it must correspond thereto.	• Must identify the animal tissue it is from.
9.42 Animal By-Product Meal (Proposed 1985, Amended 1992, Adopted 1993) IFN 5-08-786	The rendered product from animal tissues, exclusive of any added hair, hoof, horn, hide trimmings, manure, stomach and rumen contents, except in such amounts as may occur unavoidably in good processing practices. It shall not contain added extraneous materials not provided for by this definition. This ingredient definition is intended to cover those individual rendered animal tissue products that cannot meet the criteria as set forth elsewhere in this section. This ingredient is not intended to be used to label a mixture of animal tissue products.	• Catch-all of meat by-products. This ingredient is not required to disclose the animal the by-products are from. • Do not recommend feeding this to dogs.

Table 3.2. *(continued)*

Poultry

9.14 Poultry By-Products (Proposed 1963, Adopted 1964, Amended 2000) IFN 5-03-800 Poultry by-product fresh	Must consist of non-rendered clean parts of carcasses of slaughtered poultry such as heads, feet, viscera, free from fecal content and foreign matter except in such trace amounts as might occur unavoidably in good factory practice. If the product bears a name descriptive of its kind, the name must correspond thereto.	• Everything left over in the chicken except fecal matter, feathers, and foreign objects. • Not rendered.
9.10 Poultry By-Product Meal (Proposed 1985, Adopted 1990, Amended 2000) IFN 5-03-798 Poultry by-product meal rendered.	Consists of the ground, rendered, clean parts of the carcass of slaughtered poultry, such as necks, feet, undeveloped eggs, and intestines.	• Waste chicken parts ground and rendered into a meal.
9.68 Animal Digest (Proposed 1981, Amended 1983, Adopted 1990) IFN 5-06-935 Animal Digest Condensed	A material which results from chemical and/or enzymatic hydrolysis of clean and undecomposed animal tissue. The animal tissues used shall be exclusive of hair, horns, teeth, hooves and feathers, except in such trace amounts as might occur unavoidably in good factory practice and shall be suitable for animal feed. If it bears a name descriptive of its kind or flavor(s), it must correspond thereto.	• Partially digested animal protein by chemical means (hydrolysis). • May be any animal body part except hair, horns, teeth, hooves, and feathers. • Used to enhance flavor. • Usually applied to kibbles as topical liquid or coating powder.

Table 3.2. *(continued)*

Fish

51.10 Fish By-Products (Proposed 1974, Adopted 1975) IFN 5-14-509 Fish process residue fresh	Must consist of non-rendered, clean undecomposed portions of fish (such as, but not limited to, heads, fins, tails, ends, skin, bone and viscera) which result from the fish processing industry. If it bears a name descriptive of its kind, it must correspond thereto. Any single constituent used as such may be labeled according to the common or usual name of the particular portion used (such as fish heads, fish tails, etc).	• The whole fish, lips to tail.

How Dog Food Is Made

Most dry dog food is produced by extrusion, a process by which materials are heated and then pressed through a die. Today, almost all cereals, crunchy snacks and chips, baby foods, French fries, pet foods, and more are made by extrusion.

One of the critical steps in extrusion is grinding the raw materials to the correct particle size. Because most of the raw materials must be finely ground, you see a large number of "meal" ingredients on a dog food label. Extrusion requires carbohydrates to help form the finished dry kibble (gelatinization), so dry dog food packaging generally lists a carbohydrate source such as corn, wheat, or rice high on the ingredient list.

Basic Steps in Dry Dog Food Production

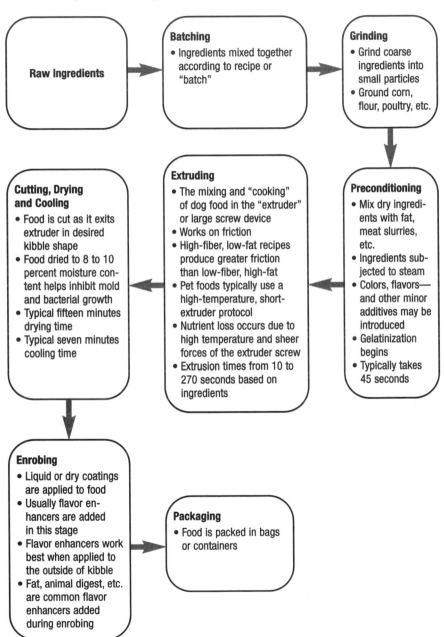

Raw Ingredients

Batching
- Ingredients mixed together according to recipe or "batch"

Grinding
- Grind coarse ingredients into small particles
- Ground corn, flour, poultry, etc.

Preconditioning
- Mix dry ingredients with fat, meat slurries, etc.
- Ingredients subjected to steam
- Colors, flavors— and other minor additives may be introduced
- Gelatinization begins
- Typically takes 45 seconds

Extruding
- The mixing and "cooking" of dog food in the "extruder" or large screw device
- Works on friction
- High-fiber, low-fat recipes produce greater friction than low-fiber, high-fat
- Pet foods typically use a high-temperature, short-extruder protocol
- Nutrient loss occurs due to high temperature and sheer forces of the extruder screw
- Extrusion times from 10 to 270 seconds based on ingredients

Cutting, Drying and Cooling
- Food is cut as it exits extruder in desired kibble shape
- Food dried to 8 to 10 percent moisture content helps inhibit mold and bacterial growth
- Typical fifteen minutes drying time
- Typical seven minutes cooling time

Enrobing
- Liquid or dry coatings are applied to food
- Usually flavor enhancers are added in this stage
- Flavor enhancers work best when applied to the outside of kibble
- Fat, animal digest, etc. are common flavor enhancers added during enrobing

Packaging
- Food is packed in bags or containers

Corn and Soy—Creating Carboholic Dogs

Making dog food out of beef, poultry, fish, whey, or lamb is expensive. To meet consumer demands for cheaper dog foods, companies have been forced to look at cheaper protein sources. Fortunately for manufacturers, much of the answer comes in the form of biggest crop in the United States: corn. Another huge U.S. crop, soybeans, helped fill in the blanks when corn was not desired. As dry dog food became popular and the extrusion process was refined, the need for starchy ingredients such as corn became even more important.

Corn and soy are good sources of dietary protein for dogs. Man has relied on these plants for thousands of years as protein providers. Many dog owners believe that dogs cannot digest or utilize corn for a variety of reasons—all of them wrong. Before you misinterpret that I recommend corn or soy as exclusive or even good protein sources for dogs, hear me out.

Many dog foods contain corn due to economics. Meat, fish, and chicken are ideal but expensive sources of protein and other essential macronutrients in dogs. Consumers have clearly demonstrated their insatiable need for cheaper dog foods, and the result is cheaper ingredients, including corn and soy as sources of dietary protein. Dog owners vote with their pocketbooks; if you want better dog food ingredients, pay for them.

Another reason for using soy and corn is convenience. In addition to being inexpensive, soy and corn are attractive to dog owners because they are easy to use and store and they resist spoilage. The extrusion process allows dog food makers to produce highly stable dry dog food that meets these needs. For a food to undergo extrusion, a starch source must be used. Corn, soy, and other starchy vegetables are nutritious ways to include starch in a dog food.

The Great Grain Debate

Many dog owners like to point out that dogs aren't designed to eat starches because they lack the enzyme amylase in the saliva. Humans have amylase in abundance, and we do well on starchy foods. This lack of salivary enzyme has nothing to do with a dog's ability to digest starches.

Dogs lack salivary amylase because they swallow their food too fast. It's a fact. Dogs have been shown to consume 100 grams or about one cup of food in an average of sixty seconds. There are several reasons for this behavior. The first is food competition. If a dog gets food into its mouth quickly, it's theirs. Therefore, fast eating is a beneficial trait. The second reason dogs eat quickly is the threat of a larger predator taking their kill or find. In other words, you'd better eat fast or someone bigger may take it from you. The third reason dogs eat quickly is because they lack large molars to efficiently chew their food. Instead, dogs tend to tear and gulp, which speeds up the consumption rate.

Because food spends little time in a dog's mouth, there is little need to secrete an enzyme to begin digestion. Instead, dogs secrete amylase in their intestinal tract where it has plenty of time to digest starches. So while there is truth to the fact that wolves or wild dogs may not eat many grains and vegetables, they can digest them.

Carbohydrates—The Truth about Grains

Carbohydrates are the body's preferred energy source because they are easily converted to simple sugars that cells need for energy. One of the first things you'll notice about a dog food label is that there is no nutritional requirement for carbohydrates. Some people mistakenly believe that this is because dogs don't require carbohydrates; they believe dogs are carnivores, which they aren't. Just because regulations don't require carbohydrates to be listed doesn't mean dogs don't need them. If you apply this same logic, you would assume that dogs don't need fiber, vitamin C, glutamine, and other nutrients. Determining how much carbohydrate a dog needs is also difficult. An active dog may perform better by eating more carbohydrates while a normal indoor lap couch potato may only get fat if it eats a high-carb diet.

Grains are a major source of carbohydrates in dog foods. Ingredients such as corn, oats, rice, wheat, and barley are commonly found in dog food. These grains contain carbohydrates, protein, vitamins and minerals, fatty acids, and fiber. Contrary to popular belief, dogs can digest and utilize grains, especially corn.

Grains contain certain fibers that promote the growth of many species of healthy bacteria in the intestinal tract (probiotics) and are a good source of many vitamins and minerals. Since

> 66 I have a great concern that the high carbohydrate content of modern dog food is contributing to, if not causing, the obesity epidemic. 99

grains contain less fat than meats, they tend to satiate a dog's appetite without adding additional fat or protein.

However, this doesn't mean carbohydrates are always good. I have a great concern that the high carbohydrate content of modern dog food is contributing to, if not causing, the obesity epidemic. Because food companies are using vegetable proteins such as corn that may also have high carbohydrate content, our dogs are eating more carbohydrates than they need. Again, corn is a good, highly digestible source of protein for dogs. The problem is that protein often comes paired with carbohydrates. Making the diets even higher in carbohydrates is the fact that dry dog food must contain starch in order to undergo extrusion and be made into the cute circles and stars dog owners seem to enjoy.

I'm often confronted with this fact when I evaluate the current diet of a weight-loss patient. For example, Cuddles was a typical six-year-old, indoor, spayed dachshund with a weight problem. When I analyzed her current diet, she was eating almost twice the calories she needed, mainly in the form of carbohydrates. Within a month of switching her to a high-protein, low-carbohydrate, low-calorie diet, she lost almost two pounds. Carb calories were killing Cuddles.

Fats in Food

Fat is one of the three major categories of food ingredients, along with proteins and carbohydrates. Fat is necessary not only for energy but also as a source of essential fatty acids, such as healthy omega-3 fatty acids. Too much fat can lead to excess weight.

Fat is also a major contributor to taste. Dogs love high-fat foods; they taste great. For this reason, dog food companies add fat to entice your dog's appetite. It is possible to override the body's normal feelings of fullness by offering a dog (or person) a delectable high-fat food, which is one of the reasons that, no matter how much you've eaten, there's always room for dessert.

That's not necessarily a good thing. When it comes to calories, fat is king. Approximately nine calories are in each gram of fat, compared to four calories in a gram of protein or carbohydrate. Thus, high-fat foods are also high-calorie. In other words, a smaller portion of a high-fat food may have more calories than a larger food portion containing mainly protein or carbohydrate.

Most fat in dog food is added fat—a separate ingredient added into the mixture. Because most of the protein sources used in commercial dog foods have been rendered, the process in which fat has been removed from protein by boiling, fat must be added to provide nutrients, flavor, and texture. On ingredient lists you commonly find this item referred to as some form of "animal fat." Sometimes fat is added in the form of an oil, such as vegetable or fish oil. Manufacturers may attempt to add descriptors to make it sound more appealing, but it's just plain fat.

For weight loss, you should look for a diet low in fat (less than 9 percent) with no added sugar and minimal flavor enhancers such as animal digests. For many dogs, canned foods are a better option because they have fewer added flavor enhancers than dry food. Dry food has twice-cooked meats (rendering and extrusion), whereas in canned dog foods the meats are typically only cooked once during extrusion, thus preserving flavor.

Controversial Additives and Flavor Enhancers

Flavor is best when the ingredients are freshest and have undergone the least processing. Modern life dictates that we usually feed our pets a commercially produced food from a bag, pouch, or can. Because of our need to balance convenience with quality ingredients, there must be some compromise. Look for a food with as few artificial or added ingredients as possible. Simple and wholesome are what your dog craves most in its food.

Yucca schidigera

Yucca schidigera is an additive beginning to appear on dog food ingredient lists. It is a cactuslike plant found in the desert regions of the southwestern United States.

Yucca schidigera is being added to pet foods as a means of reducing your dog's fecal odor. The theory is that the yucca extract, in high enough concentrations, reduces ammonia. Because some foods, especially those high in fat, contain ingredients that cause your dog's stool to have an awful smell, yucca is used to try and subdue the stench. It may also block the enzyme necessary for producing ammonia, urease. We don't yet know what, if any, effect this could have on dogs. The claims that adding yucca extract to dog foods reduces fecal odor have not be substantiated. Based on years of anecdotal evidence, yucca extract appears to be quite safe for dogs.

Ethoxyquin

One of the more controversial additives in the recent past is ethoxyquin. Ethoxyquin is a food preservative, an antioxidant that helps prevent fats from turning rancid. Ethoxyquin has been used in animal feed since 1959. In 1988, consumers began reporting adverse effects thought to be associated with ethoxyquin in several "premium" dog food brands. In 1991, the head of the FDA Center for Veterinary Medicine, Dr. David Dzanis, published a report in the *Journal of Nutrition* in response to public concern over ethoxyquin. In his journal article, Dr. Dzanis found no evidence that ethoxyquin was harmful to dogs.

Ethoxyquin has been around a long time with no proven side effects in dogs. Whenever possible, you should strive to feed your dog a food with a natural antioxidant such as Vitamin E (tocopherols). However, if the diet you know and trust contains ethoxyquin, there is no scientific evidence that you should stop it. But when in doubt, leave it out.

Reading Dog Food Labels

By now you've learned quite a bit about what goes into dog food and how those ingredients are put together. It's time to put that knowledge to work and examine a real dog food label.

Name

Naturally Complete Dog Food

What does the name mean? Not much. What's missing in the name is most important. If a dog food is made up of even 3 percent meat, poultry, or fish, the company typically includes the protein source in the name. It's simply good business. This food only tells us that it is intended for consumption by dogs, not humans. "Complete" probably indicates the food meets AAFCO nutrient requirements for all life stages.

Guaranteed Analysis

Guaranteed Analysis	
Crude Protein (Min)	25.0%
Crude Fat (Min)	12.0%
Crude Fiber (Max)	5.0%
Moisture (Max)	12.0%
Calcium (Ca) (Min)	1.1%
Phosphorus (P) (Min)	0.9%
Vitamin A (Min)	10,000 IU/kg
Vitamin E (Min)	125 IU/kg

This is a bare minimum AAFCO-required nutrient profile. This guaranteed analysis is based on the required "as fed" basis and doesn't take into account any moisture (water). In the case of this dry dog food, water accounts for 12 percent of the total product weight. If we adjust the nutrients to a dry-matter basis, the way the body uses it after the food is eaten, we find different values.

Nutrient	As Fed Percentage	Actual Percentage on Dry-Matter Basis
Crude Protein (Min)	25.0%	28.4%
Crude Fat (Min)	12.0%	13.6%
Crude Fiber (Max)	5.0%	5.7%

AAFCO Statement

Naturally Complete Dog Food is formulated to meet the nutritional levels established by the Association of American Feed Control Officials (AAFCO) Dog Food Nutrient Profiles for all life stages.

This indicates that the food is suitable for all life stages: growing puppies, pregnant or nursing females, and for maintaining the weight of adult dogs. If your dog needs to lose weight, it would not need as much fat or calories as this food includes.

Ingredient List

Ingredients

Whole-grain corn, chicken meal, beef, whole wheat, corn gluten meal, animal fat preserved with mixed-tocopherols (form of Vitamin E), soybean meal, brown rice, oat meal, pearled barley, natural flavor, calcium phosphate, calcium carbonate, caramel color, salt, potassium chloride, L-Lysine monohydrochloride, Vitamin E supplement, choline chloride, zinc sulfate, zinc proteinate, ferrous sulfate, manganese sulfate, manganese proteinate, niacin, Vitamin A supplement, copper sulfate, copper proteinate, calcium pantothenate, garlic oil, pyridoxine hydrochloride, Vitamin B-12 supplement, thiamine mononitrate, Vitamin D-3 supplement, riboflavin supplement, calcium iodate, menadione sodium bisulfite complex (source of Vitamin K activity), folic acid, biotin, sodium selenite.

The first step is to evaluate the first five ingredients, which is what the food contains the most of by weight. In this example the ingredients are whole-grain corn, chicken meal, beef, whole wheat, and corn gluten meal. Three of the five main ingredients are corn or wheat. Keep in mind that if the beef constituted at least 3 percent of the total product weight, the food could have used "with real beef" in the title. If it met the 25% Rule requirement, it could be called "Naturally Complete Beef Recipe Dog Food" or "Naturally Complete Dog Food Made with Real Beef." Those names certainly sound better.

Because the name doesn't include these AAFCO-approved terms, it is unlikely that the beef is a major part of the dog food. Because few dog owners would buy "Naturally Complete Whole Grain Corn Dog

Food," which more accurately describes this food, the manufacturer elected to omit it.

The sixth ingredient is animal fat, which is added because dogs probably wouldn't enjoy powdered chicken, corn, and wheat with a splash of beef. The good news is that the fat isn't in the top four or five ingredients. The bad news is that this food is almost exclusively carbohydrate-based.

Next you find soybean meal, brown rice, oat meal, and pearled barley. These ingredients are most likely added to aid in the extrusion process. These ingredients add some, but not much, nutritional value, so they're not a complete waste.

The next ingredient is natural flavor. In the simplest terms, a natural flavor is defined as "a substance extracted, distilled or otherwise derived from plant or animal matter, either directly from the matter itself or after it has been roasted, heated or fermented." As mentioned earlier, a natural flavor doesn't have to come from the food it is flavoring. For example, a flavor chemical derived from chicken can be used to flavor a beef dog food. In this case, we have no idea what the natural flavor is. Confusing, yes. Legal, absolutely.

The remaining ingredients are mainly added vitamins and minerals. All of these required nutrients must be added to the food because either the main ingredients—in this case, corn, chicken meal, and beef—either don't contain enough (they don't) or the processing has robbed the ingredients of these nutrients. Many dog food companies claim they add these vitamin and mineral pre-mixes to provide dogs with more nutrition than AAFCO requires. Maybe. If the whole foods already contain it in a highly digestible natural form, what's the need? Besides, these added vitamins and minerals add costs that affect the company's bottom line.

Ultimately, when it comes to your pet's health, you need to be diligent. The next chapter will help you determine how much your dog should weigh and how to get rid of any harmful pounds.

4

Rx 1:
Assess Your Dog's Weight

THE QUESTION PET OWNERS most commonly ask me is, "How much should my pet weigh?" At first this question seems deceptively simple. You would think there would be height/weight, body mass index (BMI), or similar charts that your veterinarian could use to tell you how much your pet should weigh. Unfortunately, in the world of four-legged critters, such references do not exist, which means you'll need to be a bit more creative with your assessment.

Step 1: View Your Dog from the Side

Have your pet stand up and look at it from the side. What do you see? Start at the front. Is the neck and shoulder region disproportionately large compared to your pet's head? Do you see rolls of fat and fur around the neck? Study the chest and abdomen. In lean, healthy pets, the chest should be wider than the stomach when viewed from the side. In other words, you should see a gradual upward sloping of the body as you look toward the hips. If the abdomen or stomach region hangs lower or is wider than the chest, your pet is too heavy. In fact, this is a disturbing sign because it indicates your pet may have an excess of the most dangerous type of fat present in the body, abdominal or belly fat. As you continue studying your pet from the side, look at the size of the legs relative to the body. Do they appear to be toothpicks, especially when compared to the torso? Many times, you can gauge your pet's weight and fitness by the amount of muscles and size of their legs, especially the rear legs. Too often we see plump pooches perched on precarious planks. Also note if your pet is leaning forward or backward. Most normal, healthy pets have a slight rearward slope to their body, which means they are carrying more of their weight on their larger and stronger hind legs than they are on their front legs. If your pet is shifting its weight forward, this could indicate discomfort in the knees, hips, or lower back. Some patients with severe arthritic hip or knee pain will shift almost all of their weight to the front legs.

Step 2: View Your Dog from the Rear

Study your pet from the rear as it continues to stand upright. Do you get a sense that your pet is too wide for its legs? Many times you'll see bulging at the hips and chest. A lean, healthy pet should look sleek and streamlined when viewed from the rear. Any bulging that you see should be from the upper legs, and not the hip and lower back region. If your pet looks like a hot dog on a stick, it's probably not at a healthy weight.

Step 3: View Your Dog from Above

Stand up above your pet and look down on it while it stands. Start at the head and work your way back to the tail region. Does the neck seem too wide for your pet's head? The head and neck should be at most the same width. Stocky breeds such as pugs and bulldogs may seem to have no neck. Next, look at the chest. Does it seem to be disproportionately large when compared to the size of your pet's head?

While this is certainly a judgment call, you should be able to tell if your pet's chest is too large. A tiny head attached to a broad body signals too much fat. Continue your observation rearward to the hips. Do you see a waist when viewed from above? Does your pet have a slight hourglass figure? Or do you see one large mass from shoulders to hips that gradually gets wider and wider? In people terms this would be a pear-shaped figure. Some pets have a thin chest and wide stomach region, which is perhaps the most dangerous figure to have because of the presence of intra-abdominal or belly fat. If your pet is too wide in the belly region, it's time to act quickly.

Step 4: Feel Your Pet

With your pet still standing, feel the ribs. You should be able to easily, with very little pressure applied, feel and count your pet's ribs. In very lean, muscular, and fit pets, you may even see the faint outline of three or four ribs. If you can't easily feel your pet's ribs, or if you feel a roll of fat, this is the single easiest way to tell if your pet is overweight. What about the shoulder blades? Can you feel them without applying much pressure? You should be able to feel the outline of the shoulder blades just as easily as you felt the outline of the ribs.

Next, feel your pet's stomach. Can you grab a handful of flesh? Is the belly's loose end sagging? A healthy pet will have a somewhat firm stomach with a thin layer of fat covering the abdominal muscle wall. Now feel on your pet's spine. Can you easily make out each vertebra? You should be able to feel the gentle rise and fall of each vertebra as you work your way down the spine. Do you notice rolls of fat on either side of your pet's backbone? In normal-weight pets, you should be able to feel each spine when you run your fingers down the backbone as well as the adjacent core muscles on either side of the backbone.

What about the hips? Can you feel the hip bones easily? If the hip bones are buried under mounds of fat, this indicates a problem.

Generally speaking, as a dog's body size increases, the hips become narrower.

All of this doesn't mean your pet should be bony and thin. A "walking skeleton wagging its tail" isn't a healthy weight. After all, dogs should have some fat, which is used both as an energy source and protection. What it means is that your pet should be lean and muscular. Dogs are incredibly efficient aerobic creatures. They evolved as scavengers that could travel great distances in search of food. Carrying too much extra weight put them at a disadvantage from an endurance perspective or from the ability to flee from predators at high speeds. Today's pets neither hunt for their own food nor fear being eaten. As good pet parents, we need to ensure that we maintain a healthy weight in our pet family members.

You should now have a good idea about your pet's current weight status. In the simplest of terms you should be able to determine if your pet is at a normal weight or overweight. You must be brutally honest in assessing your pet's condition. In our society, we have normalized excess weight in both ourselves and our pets. Denying there's a problem, making excuses, or even minimizing excess weight only causes further problems. This isn't about "body image" or stigma attached to being fat; this is about preserving health and preventing disease.

Calculate Your Pet's Body Condition Score (BCS)

After you've made these simple observations, you can quantify your pet's body condition. The body condition score has been widely used by veterinary health-care providers since the mid-1990s. There are basically three body-condition score scales, with each varying by the numbers used on the scale. The three most commonly used BCS ranges are a 1 to 5 scale, a 1 to 6 scale, and a 1 to 9 scale. The most important thing is not to worry over the difference between a BCS of 2 and 3 on a given scale, but rather to understand the broader context of thin and normal versus overweight and obese. Your veterinarian will use a more complex and accurate system to determine if your pet is overweight or obese and to what degree this excess weight negatively impacts your pet's health and well-being.

Here is a simplified way to assess your pet's BCS:

1 Emaciated—Too Thin: Ribs, spine, and bony protrusions are easily seen at a distance. These pets have lost muscle mass, and there is no observable body fat. Bony and starved in appearance.

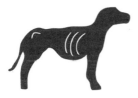
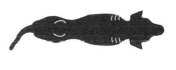

2 Thin—Normal: Ribs, spine, and other bones are easily felt. These pets have an obvious waist when viewed from above and an abdominal tuck. Lean or skinny in appearance.

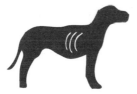
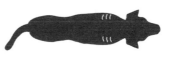

3 Normal: Ribs and spine are easily felt but not necessarily seen. There is a waist when viewed from above, and the abdomen is raised and not sagging when viewed from the side. Ideal and often muscular in appearance.

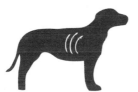
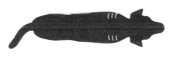

4 Overweight: Ribs and spine are hard to feel or count underneath fat deposits. Waist is distended or often pear-shaped when viewed from above. The abdomen sags when seen from the side. There are typically fat deposits on the hips, base of tail, and chest. Heavy, husky, or stout.

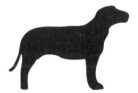
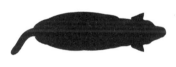

5 Obese: Large fat deposits over the chest, back, tail base, and hindquarters. The abdomen sags prominently, and there is no waist when viewed from above. The chest and abdomen often appear distended or swollen.

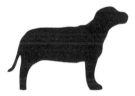
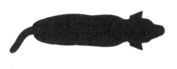

Breed Weight Charts

Another way to help determine if your pet is too heavy is to compare it to accepted breed weight ranges. While many factors can influence weight ranges, this chart offers an excellent starting point for pure-breed pets. Here is a list of some of the more popular pure breeds and normal weight ranges.

Breed	Ideal Weight Range in Pounds
Afghan hounds	58–65
Airedale terriers	40–65
Akitas	75–115
Alaskan malamutes	70–95
American Staffordshire terriers	55–65
Australian cattle dogs	30–35
Australian shepherds	40–65
Basenjis	20–25
Basset hounds	45–65
Beagles	18–30
Belgian Malinois	55–75
Bernese mountain dogs	85–110
Bichon frises	7–12
Bloodhounds	80–110
Border collies	27–45
Border terriers	11–15
Borzois	60–100
Boston terriers	10–25
Bouviers des Flandres	95–120
Boxers	50–75
Brittany spaniels	30–40
Brussels griffons	6–12
Bull terriers	Miniature: 24–32; Standard: 45–80
Bulldogs	40–50
Bullmastiffs	100–130
Cairn terriers	13–18
Cardigan Welsh corgis	25–30
Cavalier King Charles spaniels	10–18

Chesapeake Bay retrievers	55–80
Chihuahuas	4–6
Chinese cresteds	Less than 10
Chinese Shar-Peis	45–60
Chow Chows	45–70
Cocker spaniels	23–28
Collies	50–70
Dachshunds	Mini: 8–10; Standard: 10–12
Dalmatians	50–55
Doberman pinschers	65–90
English cocker spaniels	26–34
English setters	45–80
English springer spaniels	40–50
Flat-coated retrievers	60–70
French bulldogs	1922 and 22–28
German shepherds	75–95
German shorthaired pointers	45–70
German wirehaired pointers	60–70
Giant schnauzers	55–80
Golden retrievers	65–75
Gordon setters	45–80
Great Danes	110–180
Great Pyrenees	85–100
Greater Swiss mountain dogs	130–135
Havanese	7–12
Irish setters	55–75
Irish wolfhounds	90–150
Italian greyhounds	6–10 (two sizes: less than 8 or 8–10)
Japanese Chins	4–15; Two classes: under 7 and over 7
Keeshonden	Two standards: 35–45 and 55–65

Labrador retrievers	65–80
Lhasa Apsos	13–15
Maltese	4–6
Mastiffs	150–160
Miniature pinschers	8–10
Miniature schnauzers	12–15
Newfoundlands	100–150
Norwegian elkhounds	40–60
Norwich terriers	10–12
Nova Scotia duck tolling retrievers	37–50
Old English sheepdogs	60–100
Papillons	7–10
Parson Russell terriers (Jack Russell terriers)	14–18
Pekingese	Sleeve: less than 6; Mini: 6–8; Standard: 8–10
Pembroke Welsh corgis	23–27
Pomeranians	4–7
Poodles	Mini: 11–17; Standard 45–65
Portuguese water dogs	35–55
Pugs	13–18
Rhodesian ridgebacks	65–90
Rottweilers	70–135
Samoyeds	35–65
Schipperkes	12–18
Scottish terriers	18–21
Shetland sheepdogs	18–20
Shiba Inus	15–25
Shih Tzus	8–16
Siberian huskies	35–60
Silky terriers	8–11

Soft-Coated Wheaten terriers	30–45
Saint Bernards	110–200
Staffordshire bull terriers	23–38
Standard schnauzers	30–45
Tibetan terriers	20–24 (18–30 based on conformation)
Toy fox terriers	4–7
Vizslas	45–60
Weimaraners	50–70
Welsh terriers	20–21
West Highland white terriers	13–21
Whippets	25–45
Wirehaired fox terriers	13–20
Yorkshire terriers	Less than 7

When using breed weight charts, note that the individual dog's ideal weight is based on physical confirmation and not strictly on adherence to the chart. This is why there are wide weight ranges for certain breeds and genders. Dogs that are taller, wider, or longer within a breed standard may have more or less weight and still be lean and healthy. If your dog exceeds the upper limit of the weight range for its breed, this is most likely due to being overweight as opposed to being physically very large.

5

Rx 2:
Rule Out a Medical Problem

Not all dogs are overweight because they are overfed and under-exercised. The vast majority are, but you must first rule out a few medical conditions. If your dog is middle-aged or older or suddenly gains weight inexplicably, it's critically important to have your dog examined by your veterinarian before you begin a weight-loss program.

Hypothyroidism

Without a doubt, hypothyroidism, or low thyroid hormone production, is the most common disease that contributes to excess weight in dogs. Hypothyroidism most typically affects purebred middle-aged dogs, ages four to ten, but may affect dogs as young as one year old. It typically manifests in mid- to large-size breeds such as golden retrievers and cocker spaniels and is rare in toy and miniature breeds such as Chihuahuas and Pomeranians. Female dogs are more likely to develop it, too.

The most common cause of hypothyroidism, in about 95 percent of all cases, is destruction of thyroid tissue; this affliction is known as primary hypothyroidism. The two main causes of this primary hypothyroidism in dogs are immune-mediated thyroiditis and unknown atrophy or death of the thyroid tissue. Each cause accounts for about half of the cases of canine hypothyroidism. Neoplasia or cancer of the thyroid gland occurs only rarely in dogs.

One of the main causes of canine hypothyroidism, immune-mediated thyroiditis, is thought to be caused by an abnormal response of the body's immune cells in which they attack the thyroid cells. Some dog owners are concerned that vaccines play a role in the development of immune-mediated destruction of the thyroid glands, yet we know from a 2006 Purdue University study that this is not true.

Breeds predisposed to thyroiditis include:

Pointers	Maltese	Shetland sheepdogs
English setters	Beagles	Australian shepherds
Old English sheepdogs	Dalmatians	Doberman pinschers
Boxers	Golden retrievers	Cocker spaniels

The second leading cause of hypothyroidism is premature death of thyroid tissue. No one knows exactly why this occurs in some dogs. As the cells in the thyroid gland die, they are replaced with connective or fibrous tissue. In a sense, the thyroid glands begin to form nonfunctioning scar shadows of their former dynamic selves.

The clinical signs of hypothyroidism are consistent with a slowing metabolism. Most symptoms develop gradually and do not become apparent in affected dogs until at least three to five years of age.

Common Clinical Signs of Hypothyroidism in Dogs

- "Heat seekers" or cold intolerance
- Weight gain despite normal food intake
- Hair loss, especially along the sides of the body
- Dry skin and coat
- Lethargy
- Mental "dullness"
- Poor wound healing
- Increased skin infections

- Slow hair growth, may take months to regrow after grooming
- Exercise intolerance or decreased stamina
- Loss of hair on the tail, "rat tail"
- High cholesterol
- Darkly pigmented areas of skin
- Dull hair that pulls out easily

A dog displaying any of these clinical signs and that is overweight or obese should be evaluated for hypothyroidism. An overweight or obese dog without any of these clinical signs does not commonly have hypothyroidism.

While the exact reason that hypothyroidism causes obesity is still unclear, it is difficult for dogs to lose weight when they have hypothyroidism, which is why I recommend ruling out thyroid disease prior to beginning a weight-loss program. Most dogs successfully lose weight once hypothyroidism is corrected.

If a dog is overweight and has at least one clinical sign of hypothyroidism, I recommend testing for thyroid disease.

Diagnostic Tests for Hypothyroidism	Result with Hypothyroidism	
Total thyroxine (TT4)	Low	If your dog has clinical signs of hypothyroidism, low Free T4 by ED and at least 2 of the shaded tests, your dog almost certainly has Hypothyroidism
Free T4 by Equilibrium Dialysis (ED)	Low	
Thyroid-stimulating hormone (TSH)	High	
Anti-thyroglobulin antibodies	Positive	
Total cholesterol	High	
Serum chemistries	High lipase, triglycerides	
Complete blood cell count (CBC)	Anemia	

Treatment of hypothyroidism consists of daily supplementation with L-thyroxine or levothyroxine. Hypothyroid dogs should have their total thyroxine or T4 levels tested every six months. Hormonal replacement therapy in dogs should be taken very seriously and a definitive diagnosis obtained before giving something as powerful as thyroid hormone to your dog.

Cushing's Disease

Cushing's disease is fairly common in humans, horses, and dogs and contributes to weight gain in these species by a variety of mechanisms. In its most simple definition, it involves excessive production of the hormone cortisol, a naturally occurring steroid produced by the adrenal glands. Cortisol is usually referred to as the "stress hormone" because it is actively involved in the fight-or-flight response. During stress or anxiety, the adrenal glands secrete cortisol, resulting in increases in blood pressure, blood sugar, and heart and respiratory rates. Cortisol impacts many of the body's hormone-secreting organs.

About 90 percent of the time in dogs, Cushing's disease results from a benign tumor of the pituitary gland, which is called pituitary-dependent hyperadrenocorticism or PDH. The remaining 10 percent of cases are caused by a malignant tumor of the adrenal gland called adrenal tumor hyperadrenocorticism or AT.

Cushing's disease most commonly affects middle-aged and older dogs, although dogs as young as six months old have been reported with it. Breeds such as poodles, dachshunds, schnauzers, Boston terriers, and boxers have a high incidence.

One of the most reported clinical signs of Cushing's disease is an increased appetite. In fact, when treating Cushing's disease, veterinarians often watch for decreasing appetite as a sign that treatment is working.

Common Clinical Signs of Cushing's Disease in Dogs

- Increased appetite
- Potbelly abdomen; stomach appears to sag or to be swollen and distended
- Increased thirst and urination
- Chronic skin infections
- Symmetrical hair loss along the sides of body
- Thin skin, may tear easily
- Muscle weakness and loss
- Cranial cruciate ligament injuries
- Darkly pigmented areas of skin
- Calcium deposits in skin (calcinosis cutis)
- Panting
- Reproductive problems
- Neurological signs may develop with large pituitary tumors
- Anal tumors (perianal adenomas)

If your dog is overweight and has any of these clinical signs, have him evaluated by your veterinarian immediately.

Treatment of canine Cushing's disease is far from clear-cut. Several medications are available with many treatment protocols offered. Treatment should be based on your dog's specific needs and your veterinarian's recommendations, which can vary from surgery to radiation to daily medications.

Other Causes of Weight Gain

While hypothyroidism and hyperadrenocorticism are the two most common diseases that contribute to weight gain in dogs, other conditions also cause dogs to pack on the pounds.

Stress

While we don't often consider our dogs to experience stress, they do. Stress can come in the form of separation anxiety when they're left alone during the day, unusual environmental stimuli such as strange noises and odors, aggression between two pets, or lack of exercise. Stress causes overeating due to excessive secretion of the hormone cortisol. I believe stress is a major contributor to the pet obesity epidemic.

Arthritis

Excess weight can lead to osteoarthritis, but arthritis can also lead to obesity. A dog that has painful hips or elbows will be less likely to participate in aerobic activities such as walking or playing, resulting in fat accumulation if the diet is not closely controlled. Breeds that are likely to have congenital hip or elbow dysplasia include Labrador retriever, golden retriever, Belgian Malinois, Belgian shepherd, cocker spaniel, German shepherd, Rottweiler, Saint Bernard, Shetland sheepdog, Chinese Shar-Pei, and many other large-breed dogs. Keep in mind that if your dog has arthritis, decreased physical activity can lead to obesity, which worsens not only the osteoarthritis but contributes to many serious secondary conditions.

Respiratory Conditions

A dog suffering from a respiratory condition often struggles to perform even basic aerobic activities. Whenever a dog exercises less, any extra energy is stored as fat. Respiratory disease in overweight dogs is a frustrating circumstance for everyone involved. The great news is that simply maintaining a healthy weight can keep many respiratory diseases at bay. Dogs born with certain conditions or older dogs that develop breathing disorders require special attention.

One of the most common causes of respiratory-related weight gain involves brachycephalic respiratory syndrome. The term "brachycephalic" literally means "short head"; many of these dogs have a pushed-in or squashed face. Pugs, Boston terriers, Pekingese, boxers, bulldogs, Shih Tzus, and any dog with a short, flat nose, protruding or bulging eyes, and short, round face are at risk.

These dogs usually snore and snort, and otherwise have labored, noisy breathing. Because these dogs struggle to breathe, they either self-limit their activity or their owners are reluctant to exercise them because of the respiratory distress they observe during a walk or play. Either way, these dogs don't exercise enough and typically start adding pounds at a young age, further worsening their respiratory condition.

Stenotic nares (narrow nose holes) and elongated soft palate (long flap of tissue in the back of the throat) are commonly diagnosed in these breeds and can be surgically corrected. The best approach is to have these conditions corrected when your dog is young to avoid other potential respiratory complications. Dogs with brachycephalic respiratory syndrome are also prone to overheating and heat stroke.

Older dogs with respiratory diseases that limit air intake are also more likely to put on extra pounds. Any condition that limits a dog's ability to breathe will result in decreased activity. Unfortunately, many obese dogs develop respiratory diseases such as chronic-obstructive pulmonary disease (COPD) that further complicate weight loss.

Heart Disease

Heart disease causes weight gain in much the same manner as arthritis and respiratory disease—a decrease in the ability to exercise. Many dogs with heart disease develop breathing problems, further reducing their ability to go for a brisk walk. Exercise and weight reduction are critical components of the treatment of heart disease, and dogs should be encouraged to walk or participate in other low-impact activities based on your veterinarian's recommendations. Right-sided congestive heart failure can also result in the accumulation of fluid in the abdominal cavity, a condition known as ascites.

Ascites or Abdominal Fluid

Ascites is the medical term for the accumulation of fluid in the belly. If your dog's abdomen or belly begins to swell despite a normal or even decreased appetite, contact your veterinarian immediately. You may be able to feel fluid sloshing around the belly if you lightly thump it with your hand. This condition is known as an abdominal fluid wave and indicates free fluid in the abdominal cavity. The fluid that is deposited in the belly is usually the result of liver or heart disease, although many diseases can cause ascites in dogs. Treatment varies based on the cause, and has variable outcomes. Ascites needs to be treated as soon as possible before irreversible damage occurs.

Viruses

As far back as the 1980s, scientists have been studying the role that certain viruses may play in the development of obesity. The obvious interest was that if a virus caused or contributed to weight gain, then a vaccine could perhaps prevent weight gain. Unfortunately, the past thirty years have given us only insights but no solutions.

Of interest to dog lovers is the association of canine distemper virus and obesity in experiments on rats. To date, no studies connect distemper virus vaccination and weight gain in dogs.

There is growing evidence that viruses play at least some role in the worldwide human obesity epidemic. We are years away from understanding what, if any, role viruses may play in canine obesity. For now, it's too early to blame a bug for your or your pet's bulge.

The Obesity Gene

In October 1990 the U.S. National Institutes of Health (NIH) officially began the Human Genome Project, one of the most ambitious, multinational scientific endeavors in modern history. Scientists around the world would have the latest technology available to them in a race to decode human DNA within fifteen years.

That same year, the Dog Genome Project began, albeit with fewer resources and minuscule budgets. When initially completed in 2003, more than two years ahead of schedule and published on the fiftieth anniversary of the discovery of DNA, the Human Genome Project was reported to have cost $3 billion. The Dog Genome Project, when initial sequences were completed in 2005, cost approximately $30 million by comparison. If you're keeping score, that's 100 times more money spent on the Human Genome Project than on doggie DNA. The great news is that both projects are money well-spent as insights and breakthroughs are just now being realized.

In 2007, a group of British scientists identified a gene variant that may be related to human obesity. The gene, FTO (affectionately called "Fatso" by researchers), is found in about half the people of European descent and has been in existence for about 450 million years. If a person inherits two copies of the FTO variant, they are more likely to be heavier than an individual with one or no copies.

Dogs share almost 91 percent of the human FTO gene sequence, making it one of the human FTO gene's closest relatives. We currently do not understand exactly how FTO leads to obesity, only that obese people tend to have two copies of the gene. One of the proposed mechanisms is it may be involved with how the brain regulates food intake or food choices. In other words, humans or possibly dogs with two copies of the FTO gene variant may tend to overeat or favor high-calorie or high-fat foods.

Continued studies have also implicated other genes and sections of genes that may impact obesity. Regardless of an individual's genetics, lifestyle, diet, and activity play a much larger role in the development of obesity.

In other words, we are what we eat, not just our genes. The same is true for our dogs.

In a 2008 study published in the *Journal of Veterinary Internal Medicine,* researchers found that the genes associated with fat accumulation can be down-regulated or turned off by changing the diet of overweight dogs. These genes remained in the off position once the dogs lost weight. Studies such as these hold promise that our genes can be turned on or off based on diet and lifestyle.

Intestinal Microorganisms

As if viruses and genes weren't enough, new research is evaluating the role our intestinal bacteria have in contributing to obesity. The bacteria in the dog's intestine, along with diet and exercise, are critically involved in energy metabolism and obesity.

In a benchmark study on the role that gut bacteria play in energy metabolism, mice with no bacteria in their intestinal tract were given large numbers of intestinal bacteria from conventionally raised laboratory mice. Within ten to fourteen days, the previously germ-free mice gained a staggering 60 percent in body fat despite eating less than the germ-free control mice. Many reporters incorrectly interpreted this to mean that the gut bacteria made the mice fat, but the study actually demonstrated the impact gut bacteria had on metabolism and, more specifically, nutrients that lead to fat production.

We are just beginning to scratch the surface of how important intestinal microorganisms are to health. Future treatment with antibiotics, prebiotics, and probiotics may help in the fight against obesity, but more research is necessary before we can capitalize on these connections.

Medications

Certain drugs can cause your dog to gain weight. Phenobarbital (an anti-seizure medication) and steroids (prednisone, methylprednisolone, etc.) are the two most common medications associated with excess weight. Behavior-modification drugs such as Elavil (amitriptyline) and Prozac/Reconcile (fluoxetine) can lead to unwanted pounds. The high-blood pressure medication propranolol may also cause weight gain in certain dogs.

Once you've ruled out a medical problem, you can safely devise your weight loss strategy, beginning with setting realistic goals, calculating your dog's daily calories, and then choosing a weight-loss strategy.

6

Rx 3: Calculate Calories and Set Your Goals

When it comes to weight loss, the old equation of "calories in minus calories out" is as true for dogs as it is for people. The problem is that we usually don't know how many calories we should be feeding our dogs, much less how many calories we're actually feeding them. The fact is that the majority of dog owners are overfeeding their dogs by 25 to 50 percent every day because they follow the guidelines on their dog food bag. If a dog food isn't low calorie, manufacturers don't need to add a calorie statement; they can instead add a generic feeding guide to the label, which gets many dogs in trouble from a weight standpoint.

Typical Feeding Guide	
Adult Dog Size	**Feeding Amount**
3 to 12 pounds	½ to 1 cup
13 to 20 pounds	1 to 1½ cups
21 to 35 pounds	1½ to 2¼ cups
36 to 50 pounds	2¼ to 2¾ cups
51 to 75 pounds	2¾ to 3½ cups
76 to 100 pounds	3½ to 4¼ cups
Over 100 pounds	4¼ cups plus ¼ cup for each 10 pounds of body weight over 100 pounds

Remember that this dog food is formulated for all life stages. If you feed your indoor, spayed senior dog according to this guide, chances are you're feeding too much. These feeding amounts were formulated to meet the needs of active, unspayed or unneutered adult dogs. Further, this food contains higher fat and protein levels required by growing puppies and nursing mothers. This is why many dog owners commonly feed according the dog food guide and then wonder why their dogs become overweight. In order to feed your dog properly, you need to find out how many calories are in a cup or can as well as how many calories your dog needs each day.

Most dog owners are shocked at how few calories their dog actually needs. That huge "cup" of food should actually be cut in half—or at least by a third. As you begin this process, you'll need to readjust your thinking when it comes to how much you should feed your dog, beginning with learning the basics of calorie-counting.

Calories 101

Your dog requires a minimal amount of energy each day to maintain her body weight and health. This minimum amount of energy is known as the basal metabolic rate (BMR). This energy is reported as kilocalories, more commonly referred to as calories. A calorie is the amount of energy required to raise the temperature of one gram of water 1°C. For most of our dogs, BMR is close to the number of calories required to get up in the morning, go for a short walk, eat, sleep, eat, lay on couch, and sleep some more.

EYE ON THE SCIENCE

Calculating BMR

Scientists calculate BMR using complex experiments measuring body temperature, heat production, and changes in body weight and composition. As you can guess, due to difficulties in measuring these criteria and the ranges of body size and composition among different dog breeds, the results are inconsistent. In fact, ten studies on canine BMR conducted from 1926 to 1986 ranged in their findings from 48–88 to 78–114 kcal ME·kg $BW^{-0.75}$. That's a huge range in the number of recommended daily calories.

If you want to gauge your dog's calorie needs, there are two formulas you can use, the first of which works best for active adult dogs.

In 1993, Zentek and Meyer derived a useful formula for calculating energy requirements in adult dogs: *kilocalories = 358 + (39 X body weight in kilograms)*. To convert your dog's weight in pounds to kilograms, simply divide the number of pounds by 2.2 (pounds / 2.2 = kilograms). This formula works well for active adult dogs. For spayed or neutered dogs, reduce the number of kilocalories (or "calories" for all of us nonscientists) by 25 to 30 percent. Dogs older than five to seven years of age may decrease the number of calories by an additional 10 to 15 percent. Indoor, inactive dogs may also require fewer calories.

Zentek and Meyer's formula is still widely used, although the formula that veterinarians most often use today is *kilocalories = (30 X body weight in kilograms) + 70*. This represents the dog's Resting Energy Requirements (RER), or the number of calories your dog needs to maintain normal physiological requirements. It is not intended as a guideline for active dogs. For most urban, sedentary, neutered indoor dogs, RER is generally an adequate number of calories to maintain a lean, healthy weight. Remember that the key link to energy requirements is your dog's activity level. More active, energetic dogs require more calories. Sedentary dogs that spend the majority of their days indoors require fewer calories as do older dogs and those that are spayed and neutered.

Calorie Chart				
Typical Total Daily Calories to Achieve Weight Loss in Adult Spayed or Neutered Dogs				Maintenance Diet for Adult Spayed or Neutered Dogs
Ideal or Target Weight (lbs)	RER to Feed for Weight Loss (kcals per day)	80% RER (kcals per day)	70% RER (kcals per day)	(kcals per day)
5	138	111	97	166
6	152	121	106	182
7	165	132	116	199
8	179	143	125	215
9	193	154	135	231
10	206	165	144	248
11	220	176	154	264
12	234	187	164	280
13	247	198	173	297
14	261	209	183	313
15	275	220	192	329
16	288	231	202	346
17	302	241	211	362
18	315	252	221	379
19	328	263	230	395
20	343	274	240	411
21	356	285	249	428
22	370	296	259	444
23	384	307	269	460
24	397	318	278	477

Calorie Chart (continued)				
Ideal or Target Weight (lbs)	**RER to Feed for Weight Loss** (kcals per day)	**80% RER** (kcals per day)	**70% RER** (kcals per day)	**Maintenance Diet** (kcals per day)
25	411	329	288	493
26	425	340	297	509
27	438	351	307	526
28	452	361	316	542
29	465	372	326	559
30	479	383	335	575
31	493	394	345	591
32	506	405	354	608
33	520	416	364	624
34	534	427	374	640
35	547	438	383	657
36	561	449	393	673
37	575	460	402	689
38	588	471	412	706
39	602	481	421	722
40	615	492	431	739
41	629	503	440	755
42	643	514	450	771
43	656	525	459	788
44	670	536	469	804
45	684	547	479	820
46	697	558	488	837
47	711	569	498	853
48	725	580	507	869
49	738	591	517	886
50	752	601	526	902
51	765	612	536	919

Calorie Chart *(continued)*

Ideal or Target Weight (lbs)	RER to Feed for Weight Loss (kcals per day)	80% RER (kcals per day)	70% RER (kcals per day)	Maintenance Diet (kcals per day)
52	779	623	545	935
53	793	634	555	951
54	806	645	564	968
55	820	656	574	984
56	834	667	584	1000
57	847	678	593	1017
58	861	689	603	1033
59	875	700	612	1049
60	888	711	622	1066
62	915	732	641	1099
64	943	754	660	1131
66	970	776	679	1164
68	997	798	698	1197
70	1025	820	717	1229
72	1052	841	736	1262
74	1079	863	755	1295
76	1106	885	774	1328
78	1134	907	794	1360
80	1161	929	813	1393
85	1229	983	860	1475
90	1297	1038	908	1557
95	1365	1092	956	1639
100	1434	1147	1004	1720
105	1502	1201	1051	1802
110	1570	1256	1099	1884
115	1638	1311	1147	1966
120	1706	1365	1194	2048

Some Calorie Caveats

When discussing weight loss and reducing calories in dogs, we must be certain to exclude dogs that are pregnant, lactating, or growing. Young, pregnant, or nursing dogs should not be placed on a weight-loss program.

It's also important to point out that you can't simply put your dog on a diet by feeding him less food because when you cut the portion size, you also cut nutrients. This is why specially-formulated weight-loss diets are often preferred (see chapter 7 for my recommendations). By feeding your dog a weight-loss formula, your dog will get fewer calories while maintaining optimal nutrition. A diet does not mean starvation.

Getting Started

Before you begin a weight-loss program, you need to check with your vet to make sure your dog is healthy enough. Embarking on a diet plan with a dog that has a subclinical medical problem (one that isn't displaying any clinical signs yet) can lead to serious consequences.

The Step Weight-Loss Plan

Once your veterinarian has declared your dog healthy to begin a diet, you need to set goals for safe weight loss. A general rule of thumb is that your dog should be able to lose approximately 3 to 5 percent of her body weight per month. That means an 80-pound dog that needs to lose 15 pounds can lose 2.5 to 4 pounds per month. Safe and gradual weight loss helps preserve muscle mass and avoid potential nutritional deficiencies. Further, this plan allows you as a pet owner to alter your dog's lifestyle and encourage activity, play, and changes in diet and treats. Many dogs initially experience tremendous weight loss during the first three months, and then the rate decreases over time. This response is normal and does not indicate that you are doing anything wrong.

The safest and most successful way to help your dog lose weight is to pursue small goals over time. We call this a stair-step weight-loss plan. Think of a flight of stairs. The goal is to get one from one floor to the next. In this example, your starting floor is your dog's present weight, and your ending floor is your dog's ideal weight. While there are many ways to move from one floor to another, the safest and surest way is to take a series of steps that lead you to your goal. Too often, dog owners want to take a speedy elevator ride, but quick fixes more often than not result in only temporary improvements, as opposed to a lifetime of healthy habits. Patience, perseverance, and discipline are required to make meaningful changes. By attaining a series of small goals, you'll discover that lifestyle changes are easier to accomplish.

So how long does this process take? While no one answer applies to every situation, most dogs should be able to reach their ideal weight in six to twelve months. Healthy dogs that are able to exercise more vigorously may see results faster. Older dogs or those with arthritis or other medical conditions may require more time. In general, dogs that need to lose less than 30 percent of their body weight should reach their ideal or normal weight within six months. For dogs that need to lose more than 30 percent of their current body weight, the time period may be extended to nine to twelve months.

Figure 6.1. Step Weight-Loss Plan

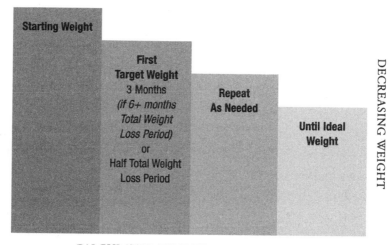

CALCULATED TIME TO IDEAL WEIGHT

Let's consider an example to demonstrate how to calculate your pet's weight loss over time.

Harley, an Obese Dachshund

Harley is a seven-year-old dachshund in trouble. Tipping the scales at 22 pounds, he is 10 pounds overweight, which places him squarely in the obese category—80 percent over his ideal weight. His veterinarian has performed a physical examination and the recommended blood and urine tests, and found Harley to be in good health with the exception of early osteoarthritis.

Harley's ideal weight is determined to be 12 pounds. If we were simply to feed him the number of calories a 12-pound dog should receive, we would risk serious physiological damage. Morbidly obese dogs are also at risk for developing a serious liver complication called hepatic lipidosis. This is why you should never start your obese pet on a weight-loss program without consulting your veterinarian first.

To apply this step weight-loss program to Harley's situation, take the number of pounds he needs to lose to reach his ideal weight—in this case, 10 pounds. Since Harley is morbidly obese with some physical complications, plan on a twelve-month period for weight loss. Harley needs to lose about 1 pound per month to reach his target within a year.

Next, break up Harley's weight-loss goals into several steps over the next twelve months. The halfway step will be in six months, at which time Harley should be at approximately 17 pounds. In the first three months, he should lose 3 pounds and attain his first target weight of 19 pounds. The steps are taken and recalculated every three months until his ideal weight is achieved.

Figure 6.2. Harley's Step Weight-Loss Plan

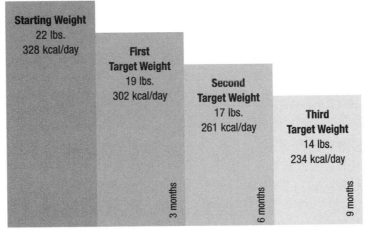

Harley's initial caloric guidelines will be based on this first target weight. Using the formula presented earlier, we calculate Harley's desired initial caloric intake:

RER = [(first target weight in pounds ÷ 2.2) x 30] + 70
RER = [(19 ÷ 2.2) x 30] + 70
RER = (8.6 x 30) + 70
RER = 258 + 70
RER = 328 kilocalories or calories per day

Because the body quickly learns to adapt to changes in caloric intake, we closely monitor Harley's weight, typically every thirty days. Some dogs adapt quickly to changes in caloric intake, and you must restrict calories or increase activity sooner. Other dogs may remain on a more constant caloric content throughout the entire weight-loss period. Some dogs may even do better on a diet with a different composition of fats, proteins, and carbohydrates, as discussed later.

In Harley's case, at three months he weighs 18.6 pounds. It's time to step down the number of calories. Our next target weight is 17 pounds at six months.

RER = (second target weight in kg x 30) + 70
RER = [(17 ÷ 2.2) x 30] + 70
RER = (7.72 x 30) + 70
RER = 232 + 70
RER = 302 kilocalories or calories per day

Harley's owner continues to follow through exceptionally well, and in six months Harley has slimmed down to 16 pounds—only 4 pounds more until he reaches his ideal weight of 12 pounds. Then we recalculate the number of calories based on our nine-month target weight of 14 pounds.

RER = (third target weight in kg X 30) + 70
RER = [(14 ÷ 2.2) X 30] + 70
RER = (6.36 X 30) + 70
RER = 191 + 70
RER = 261 kilocalories or calories per day

At nine months Harley's progress slowed down. He didn't quite meet his target of 14 pounds. Instead, the scales revealed 15.2 pounds. Harley's owner is understandably upset. He has been strictly adhering to the feeding guideline, although he owns up to giving Harley a few extra treats here and there. Harley's owner has a decision to make. Whenever a dog fails to reach a target weight within three months, something has to change. Harley's owner has four options:

1 Reduce the number of calories being fed per day (maximum 70 percent RER unless instructed by veterinarian).
2 Change the type of food he's feeding (see chapters 7 and 8).
3 Increase exercise (see chapter 9).
4 Use prescription drugs (see chapter 12).

Harley's owner expresses that he is unsure if he can further reduce the calories. He's pleased that Harley enjoys the food and is reluctant to change it. He's uncomfortable resorting to medications, because Harley has done so well thus far. Therefore, the safest and easiest way to get back on track is to increase Harley's physical activity. The good news is that since Harley has lost weight, he's able to jump into the car without help, and seems spryer during their morning and evening walks. The plan is to increase the morning walk by fifteen minutes for a total of thirty-five to forty minutes and increase the evening walk by fifteen minutes to thirty-five minutes total. Additionally, Harley's owner plans to increase the pace to a brisker walk, as opposed to their leisurely stroll.

RER = (target weight in kg x 30) + 70
RER = [(12 ÷ 2.2) x 30] + 70
RER = (5.45 x 30) + 70
RER = 164 + 70
RER = 234 kilocalories or calories per day

Harley is scheduled to return to the veterinarian for weigh-ins every three to four weeks during this final stage of his step weight-loss plan. If Harley doesn't lose weight, we may change our approach. The last 5 to 10 percent of weight loss is often the most challenging for dogs. Lean muscle mass is being created at this time, and abdominal fat is being reduced. Most dogs require an increase in physical activity during the final stage of their weight-loss plan to reach their ideal weight. Dogs are naturally lean creatures with long muscles and relatively light skeletal mass. To achieve the desired level of fitness, dogs need to return to the largely aerobic lifestyles from which they evolved. Dogs that are indoors most of the time have difficulty developing the strong muscles and support tissues required for an ideal healthy body composition without structured daily exercise.

As Harley's owner increases their physical activity, Harley lost the last remaining pounds. Less than eleven months into this step weight-loss plan, Harley achieves his ideal weight of 12 pounds. Harley's owner barely recognizes his dog. Harley is eager to get up in the morning for their brisk walks and he loves riding in the car. Now he can jump into his seat without assistance, and the aches and pains of arthritis are all but gone. Harley's risk for paralysis is almost nonexistent.

Boris, an Overweight Golden Retriever

Boris is a five-year-old neutered male golden retriever who has put on a few pounds in the past two years. Boris had remained a constant 72 pounds until his owners became ill, causing them to reduce their daily walks to less than fifteen minutes per day. Boris has gained 6 pounds in the past year and a half to weigh in at 78 pounds. Boris is beginning to have difficulty rising after he lies in one place for more than a couple of hours and he navigates more cautiously than before on the flight of stairs that leads to their bedroom. Boris's owner is concerned that if he can't walk up the stairs, she won't be able to help him due to her own frail health. Boris's veterinarian concludes that he is healthy enough to begin a weight-loss program.

As Boris is a relatively young adult and is not classified as obese, his weight-loss plan should be of short duration. If Boris is able to exercise more while reducing calories, he should be able to lose 6 pounds within three to five months. In situations where an owner is unable to exercise her dog enough for weight-loss goals, a dog walker or friendly neighbor comes in handy. In cases where increasing physical activity is impractical, more careful attention must be placed on the diet. Boris's owner has a neighbor who agrees to take Boris for one brisk thirty-minute walk per day, weather permitting.

Figure 6.3. Boris's Step Weight-Loss Plan

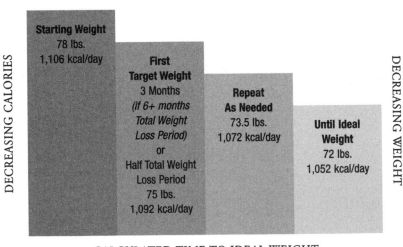

DECREASING CALORIES

Starting Weight
78 lbs.
1,106 kcal/day

First
Target Weight
3 Months
(if 6+ months
Total Weight
Loss Period)
or
Half Total Weight
Loss Period
75 lbs.
1,092 kcal/day

Repeat
As Needed
73.5 lbs.
1,072 kcal/day

Until Ideal
Weight
72 lbs.
1,052 kcal/day

DECREASING WEIGHT

CALCULATED TIME TO IDEAL WEIGHT

Boris's owner pays close care to his feedings and treats, and within two months Boris achieves his ideal weight. Because Boris's energy levels have increased, the neighbor agrees to continue with their daily walks. If Boris misses his daily walk, his owner makes sure she reduces his calories by a treat or two.

You Must Track Your Treats

For a weight-loss program to be successful, you must take into account the number of calories that your dog's treats contain. Treats are the silent saboteurs of good weight-loss plans. Many dog owners feed the correct amount of calories from their main diet, yet destroy their efforts with too many high-calorie treats. The adage, "a calorie is a calorie" applies to dogs as well as people. Even though treats are bite-size morsels, they pack a caloric punch. For many dogs, even two to three treats a day on top of a healthy diet is enough to equal pounds over a year's time. The following charts show the effects those little treats can have on your dog in human terms. The results might surprise you. In general, for your dog's diet to be successful, you need to beware of the biscuits.

10-pound Dog *Requiring 200 to 220 Calories Per Day*			
If Your Dog Eats This . . .	**Number of Calories**	**It's Like You Eating That . . .**	**Number of Calories**
1 The Good Life Recipe Wholesome Bone—mini	62	3 Hershey's Milk Chocolate Bars	690
1 Biscuit—Milk-Bone Gravy Bones for Small and Medium Size Dogs	45	2 Krispy Kreme Chocolate Iced Glazed Doughnuts	500

10-pound Dog *(continued)*			
1 Blue Dog Bakery Peanut Butter and Molasses—Small	39	27 Cadbury's Mini Eggs	427
1 Purina Beggin' Strip	30	1 McDonald's Cheeseburger	310
1 Snausages	25	1 McDonald's Hamburger	260
1 Greenies Teenie	25	2 12-oz. Coke Classics	280
1 Pup-Peroni	24	1 Little Debbie Fudge Brownie	270

Based on a 2300 calories-per-day human diet

20-pound Dog
Requiring 340 to 360 Calories Per Day

If Your Dog Eats This ...	Number of Calories	It's Like You Eating That ...	Number of Calories
1 Purina Busy Bone Chew Treat Dental for Small/Med Dogs	277	3 McDonald's Chocolate Triple Shake – 16 oz.	1740
1 The Good Life Recipe Wholesome Bone—Small/Medium	276	7½ Hershey Milk Chocolate Bars	1725
1 Snausages SnawSomes Peanut Butter and Apple Flavor	137	½ Large Domino's Pizza with Extra Cheese (4 slices, 14")	916
1 Small Pedigree Denta-Bone	105	Denny's Buttermilk Pancake Platter (3 pancakes)	660
Healthy Treats for dogs Dental Wellness	54	2 Cheese Krystal cheeseburgers	320
1 Purina Healthy Weight (Turkey and Rice) treat	26	1 4-piece McNuggets	170

20-pound Dog *(continued)*			
1 Meaty Bone Biscuit— Small	27	2 Keebler E.L. Fudge Double Stuffed Sandwich cookies	180
1 Greenies Light—Petite	51	1 McDonald's Hot Fudge Sundae	330

Based on a 2300 calories-per-day human diet

40-pound Dog			
Requiring 620 to 650 Calories Per Day			
If Your Dog Eats This . . .	**Number of Calories**	**It's Like You Eating That . . .**	**Number of Calories**
1 Purina Busy Bone— Small/Medium	309	4 McDonald's Egg McMuffins	1200
1 Good Life Wholesome Bone—Small	276	4 Chocolate Éclairs	1048
1 Premium Pig Ear	231	6 12-oz. Coke Classics	840
1 Dingo Meat In The Middle—Small bone	176	2 Taco Bell Taco Supremes and 1 20-oz. Coke	673
1 Snausages SnawSomes Peanut Butter and Apple Flavor	137	1 Burger King Large French Fries	500
1 Regular Greenies Dental Chew	90	1 Hot Pockets Meatball and Mozzarella	330
1 Nutro Weight Management Biscuit	49	1 bag Sugar Babies (30 pieces)	180
1 Waggin' Train Meat Blast	40	1 chocolate cupcake	131

Based on a 2300 calories-per-day human diet

60-pound Dog
Requiring 890 to 950 Calories Per Day

If Your Dog Eats This ...	Number of Calories	It's Like You Eating That ...	Number of Calories
1 Purina Busy Bone Chew Treat Ultimate Chew Chew Treat Meaty Middle for Medium Dogs	700	2 Burger King Original Whoppers with Cheese and Small French Fries	1750
1 Good Life Wholesome Bone—Large	552	4 Kentucky Fried Chicken Original Recipe chicken breasts	1480
1 SteakChew Long-lasting Chew Snack	383	1 Long John Silver's Fish Sandwich, 1 Regular Fries, 1 20-oz. Coke Classic	948
Dingo Meat in the Middle— Medium	280	2 slices Domino's Brooklyn Pepperoni and Extra Cheese pizza (large pizza)	658
1 Milk-Bones Large Dog Biscuit	120	1 Snickers Bar	280
2 Dogswell Happy Hips Glucosamine and Chondroitin—Lamb and Rice treats	74	1 4-Piece McNuggets	170
1 Blue Dog Bakery Live Well Super Premium Treats—Medium	66	3 Pepperidge Farm Milk Chocolate Milano cookies	170
1 Nutro Ultra Senior Dog Biscuits	50	1 Little Debbie Devil Squares Cakes	135

Based on a 2300 calories-per-day human diet

80-pound Dog			
Requiring 1200 to 1500 Calories Per Day			
If Your Dog Eats This . . .	**Number of Calories**	**It's Like You Eating That . . .**	**Number of Calories**
Hartz Dentist's Best with Dental Shield—Chew Treats (For large dogs over 55 pounds)	1060	34 Chips Ahoy chocolate chip cookies (160 kcals per 3 cookies)	1806
1 Beggin' Chew—Large	672	1 Wendy's Classic Single Hamburger with Everything, 1 medium fry, 1 20-oz. Coke Classic	1158
1 Blue Buffalo Health Bar with Bacon, Egg and Cheese	108	1 Starbucks Caffe Mocha with Skim Milk (16 oz.)	180
1 Large DentaBone	300	1 Thick Vanilla Milk Shake (16 oz.)	509

Based on a 2300 calories-per-day human diet

7

Rx 4: Choose the Best Commercial Diet

The science of nutrition is inexact. We are still in the infancy of understanding the myriad ways that food affects our health and well-being. For example, nutritionists have yet to describe an ideal diet for humans, despite intensive research and incredible funding. To think we have all the answers for dog nutrition is not only cavalier but also dangerous. Nutrition is an extremely complex subject in which we are far from completely understanding. Therefore when clients ask me, "What should I feed my dog?" I don't have a single recommendation that works for every dog. Rather, I believe owners should select food based on their dogs' needs and preferences, and how the dog and owner live in the real world. In a perfect world in which we all ate a truly wholesome and balanced diet, you and your dog would share dinner. Fresh meats, fish, poultry, and eggs combined with fresh vegetables and grains would add nutrition in a delicious fashion. Unfortunately, few of us live in that world, and home cooking may not work for everyone due to time constraints, cost considerations, and concerns over calculating proper calories and nutrients. To balance our hectic lifestyles with optimal nutrition and weight-loss objectives, I typically recommend what I call a Hybrid Menu, which means that you supplement a commercial diet food by preparing your dog's meals two to three times a week (see chapter 8 for details). If preparing your dog's meals seems far-fetched or too time-consuming for you, don't fret. There are many nutritious and highly effective commercial weight-loss diets available. The key is finding the one that works best for your dog.

Recommended Commercial Weight-Loss Diets

Ranking food is risky business. In reality, what's best for one dog may be wholly unsuitable for another. Making things more complicated is the fact that dog foods constantly tinker with their formulations, resulting in "this year's best" becoming "next year's worst" with little, if any, warning.

In compiling a list of recommended weight-loss diets, I've tried to use brands that have a long history and good quality control, based on my own personal experience. Inclusion on these lists doesn't mean a diet will work for your dog nor does exclusion indicate a diet will fail. Ultimately the choice of a weight-loss diet must include your veterinarian's recommendation, your dog's medical history and preferences, your preferred weight-loss strategy, and palatability. Palatability is critical, because if your dog doesn't like it, he won't eat it.

Regardless of the weight-loss approach or brand of food you choose, I recommend a diet that contains ideally less than 250 kcals per cup or can, but I'll consider a diet containing about 300 kcals per cup or can. If you feed a diet with many more calories per cup or can and you have a dog that should weigh less than 40 pounds, you'll find you must feed very small amounts in order to achieve the reduced number of calories. This leads to your dog feeling less satisfied and a greater likelihood you'll make a measuring mistake. Additionally, if you feed too little of a maintenance (normal) food, you may inadvertently rob your dog of essential nutrients. For these reasons, I advocate specially formulated weight-loss diets instead of feeding less of your regular dog food. Plenty of excellent, wholesome diets are available; the problem is that they contain too many calories for practical weight reduction. When it comes to weight loss, calories are king. When it comes to low-calorie diets, many of the best are available from your veterinarian or specialty pet food retailer.

Another often overlooked matter in food selection is quality control. I tend to recommend larger, well-known brands. These large pet food manufacturers have the resources to directly oversee their products and often have better control of their ingredient sources. After the 2007 pet food recall, most of the major brands improved their quality-control procedures, and government oversight of nationally distributed brands tightened. That being said, even the biggest brands can stumble. There are also many emerging boutique brands that produce excellent dog foods, albeit in fewer varieties and at a premium price. Stay alert to any food recalls or investigations, and make your selections accordingly. Use these lists as a starting point in conjunction with your veterinarian's advice.

High-Protein Weight-Loss Diets

I typically start my patients with a diet containing at least 30 percent protein on a dry-matter basis (DMB).

Diet	Kcals per cup
Royal Canin Veterinary Diet Canine Calorie Control CC 32 High Protein Dry Food	234
Purina Veterinary Diets OM Overweight Management Canine Formula Dry	266
Acana Light & Fit	325

Balanced Protein-Carbohydrates Diets

Balanced protein-carbohydrate diets are typically low in fat. Some of these diets are described as "high protein," but anything less than 30 percent protein content does not meet my definition of "high protein." These diets work very well in most dogs.

Diet	Kcals per cup
Iams Veterinary Formula Weight Loss Restricted Calorie Dry Dog Food	217
Purina Veterinary Diets—Small Bites DH Canine Formula	302
Artemis Company Artemis Fresh Mix Weight Management	308
Purina Veterinary Diets—Regular Bites DH Canine Formula	315
California Natural Low-Fat Rice & Lamb Meal Adult Dry Dog Food	317
Wellness Super 5 Mix Weight Management Dry Dog Food	325
BLUE Buffalo Longevity for Mature Dogs	330
Merrick Senior Medley	337

High-Fiber Weight-Loss Diets

High-fiber diets generally have approximately 20 percent fiber or more. Remember that higher fiber often means more bathroom duty for many dogs.

Diet	Kcals per cup
Royal Canin Veterinary Diet Canine Calorie Control CC 26 High Fiber	231
Hill's Prescription Diet r/d Canine Dry Food	242
Hill's Prescription Diet w/d Canine Dry Food	243

Vegetarian Diet

For dog owners choosing a nonmeat weight-loss approach, be sure to closely watch the calories in your dog's food. Many vegetarian and vegan diets contain a high number of calories due to the reliance on carbohydrate sources for proteins and other essential nutrients. A vegetarian or vegan diet is appropriate for most dogs suffering from food allergies or for vegetarian and vegan owners.

Diet	Kcals per cup
AvoDerm Natural Vegetarian Adult Dog Food	324

How to Pick a Premium Diet

Most dog owners feed their pet from a bag or can for a variety of reasons. This is perfectly fine if you select the food wisely.

First, *choose a protein* source that you and your dog prefer. Make sure the protein source is the first listed ingredient and that it isn't a "meal" or "by-product." I prefer fish sources followed by turkey and poultry. Your dog can still lose weight on a beef-based diet; fish and fowl are just my personal preferences as I look for ways to reduce my dog's impact on the environment.

Next, *choose a brand you trust.* Trust in the pet food industry was badly shaken after the 2007 pet food recall. I typically recommend a nationally distributed brand because of the additional FDA oversight. Pet foods sold across state lines come under federal jurisdiction, and I prefer that added layer of security, however thin.

Select a carbohydrate blend that suits your dog well. Some dogs have wheat allergies, so I recommend avoiding wheat grains whenever possible. If your dog tolerates corn well, I have no objections to a diet with corn, based on current research. Avoid any food with carbohydrates as its first ingredient, unless the diet is vegetarian.

Evaluate the caloric density or **weight-loss approach of the foods you're considering.** Weight-loss foods typically follow one of three approaches:

1 "Filler Formula"—high in fiber, low in calories.

2 "Dogkins Diet"—high in protein and possibly fiber, low in carbs (see Premium Protein on page 123).

3 "Low Balanced"—a low-calorie, protein-carbohydrate balanced diet (see Quelling Carbohydrate Confusion on page 127).

Each of these weight-loss strategies works for dogs in general, but not every one works for every dog. I generally begin with a high-protein, low-carb diet and then change in three months if the patient fails to lose significant weight. High-protein diets tend to better satisfy even the biggest beggars than other approaches in my experience. Whichever approach you favor, here are some other things to watch for:

Avoid added sugar. If you see "glucose," "dextrose," "sucrose," "high-fructose corn syrup," "maltodextrins," or similar sugar additives, don't buy it. Sugar is added only to enhance palatability, regardless of what the packaging claims. (Recently some dog food companies have added honey as a "prebiotic." Clever.)

Avoid excessive preservatives. All packaged dog food requires some preservative to maintain freshness and prevent rancidity. An example of a safe preservative is tocopherol or Vitamin E. Preservatives such as butylated hydroxyanisole (BHA) and butylated hydroxytoluene (BHT) should be avoided as much as possible. While research is inconclusive on the potential negative health impacts of BHA and BHT, large doses have been shown to cause tumors in laboratory mice.

Be wary of artificial colorings and flavors. Ask why food needs artificial flavors and colorings. What needs to be covered up or altered? If you see FD&C Yellow No. 5, beef flavor, and related ingredients, try another dog food.

You usually get what you pay for when it comes to healthier dog food. Be prepared to pay significantly more for a premium diet than the low-cost grocery store brand, especially one with high protein. The most expensive food isn't necessarily the best, though. Do your homework; you also may save a few bucks while feeding your dog a superior food.

Dog foods constantly change. I encourage my clients to remain open-minded when it comes to brand selection. Just because a dog food was superior in the past doesn't mean it's the best choice today. Just because a breeder or neighbor has good results doesn't mean your dog will. Keep up with nutritional research, and don't hesitate to try different approaches over time. Don't be afraid to mix things up when it comes to your dog's diet. The most important thing to understand when it comes to diets is that *no one diet is for every dog*. The same is true for people, which explains why bookstores carry literally dozens of books on weight loss and diet. While no one perfect diet food or program works for all dogs, you can follow some general guidelines to assess if the food is right for your dog or if it's time for a change.

Calorie Content

If you are feeding your dog a commercial dog food, the first step in evaluating the dog's current diet is to determine how many calories are in a cup or can. As explained earlier, AAFCO and the FDA do not require pet food manufacturers to include this information on the label. Some dog foods list the number of calories in terms of calories per cup or can, and others include calories per kilogram. If your food lists the number of calories per kilogram, you'll need to do some math or contact the company for this information. To convert calories per kilogram into calories per cup, follow these steps:

1 Find on the label a statement such as "3704 kcal/kg of metabolizable energy (ME) on an as fed basis (calculated)." This statement means the food has 3704 calories per kilogram.
2 Weigh a 1-cup measuring container.
3 Add 1 cup of the dog food and weigh the cup and food together.
4 Subtract the weight of food plus cup from the empty measuring cup. This is the weight of the food.
5 Divide the weight of the food by 35.3 (1 kg is equal to 35.3 ounces). This calculation gives you the number of kilograms in a cup.
6 Multiply the number of kilograms in a cup by the number of kilocalories in kilogram.
This gives you the number of calories per cup.

Let's use an example:

1 You have a food that contains 3704 calories per kilogram.
2 Measuring cup weighs 4 ounces.
3 Measuring cup and 1 cup of food weigh 8 ounces.
4 1 cup of food therefore weighs 4 ounces.
5 4 ÷ 35.3 = 0.113.
6 0.113 x 3704 = 420 calories per cup

Once you determine the number of calories in your present dog food, you need to decide how much to feed your dog. The answer is more complicated than just calories, but you can draw some conclusions based on the caloric content of what you're feeding.

You want to choose a dog food that contains relatively few calories per cup. Your dog can thus eat more and feel "fuller." Over the years, a variety of strategies have been used to make diet dog food more filling: puffing the kibble up with air (zero calories!) to make it larger, adding indigestible fiber (also with no calories but can wreak havoc on the bowels), changing the texture of the food to encourage more chew-

> ❝ In general, a weight-loss dog food should contain less than 250 calories per cup. Whenever possible, try to select a food in the 210 to 230 calories per cup range. ❞

ing, and so on. Some have worked better than others and persist in the marketplace. Others are abandoned quickly (you can only puff up kibbles so big before they pop—or cause choking). In general, a weight-loss dog food should contain less than 250 calories per cup. Whenever possible, try to select a food in the 210 to 230 calories per cup range.

Fat Content

It's hard to formulate a low-calorie-density dog food that contains a lot of fat. AAFCO requires any "low fat" dry dog food to contain less than 9 percent fat. That's a pretty decent amount since the AAFCO minimum for adult maintenance diets is 5 percent. Ideally, a dry diet would contain 5 to 9 percent fat. But before you take the label's word for it, you'll need to do a little fact checking.

Recommended Calorie and Fat Content for Weight Loss in Neutered Adult Dogs			
Calorie range per cup or can (kcals)	Ideal calories per cup or can (kcals)	Fat percentage range	Ideal fat percentage
200 to 300 kcals	210 to 230	7 to 12%	5 to 9%

FAT FACT CHECK

Examine the following example of a low-fat dog food label:

Crude fat not less than	6.5%
Crude fat not more than	7.0%
Moisture not more than	78.0%

First of all, exactly how much fat is in this food?

Let's assume the food contains 7 percent fat. I always recommend you use the higher number in a range because that is probably closer to the truth than the lower number due to moisture content.

Because this diet contains 78 percent moisture, we need to subtract the water content from the food since the water contains no fat.

Fat content of food on a dry-matter basis = Percentage fat as
    fed/amount of dry matter x 100
Fat = 7% as fed
Dry matter = 100% − 78% = 22%
7 ÷ 22 = 0.318
0.318 x 100 = 32% fat on a dry-matter basis

The food actually contains 32 percent fat on a dry-matter basis! Keep in mind that the higher the moisture content of a food, the higher the percentage a nutrient will be on a dry-matter basis. Look at the following chart to see the impact of moisture content on nutrient percentage when viewed on a dry-matter basis:

7% Fat on Label—"As Fed"	
Moisture content	Percentage fat on dry-matter basis
10%	8%
20%	9%
65%	20%
78%	32%
85%	47%

Evaluate the amount of fat your current dog food contains. In general terms, canned foods will have higher fat and protein content than dry foods. If it's above 12 percent fat "as fed," it's probably too high to help your dog lose weight. Besides, those calories end up somewhere, usually in the form of dangerous white adipose tissue or belly fat.

Eating excess fat causes the body to look for anywhere to store it—and fast. High-fat meals cause your body to store fat around vital organs instead of in the abdomen as it normally does. Unfortunately, organs such as the heart, liver, and pancreas are the first choices, leading to metabolic syndrome, insulin resistance, and heart and liver disease.

> “ Evaluate the amount of fat your current dog food contains. If it's above 12 percent fat "as fed," it's probably too high to help your dog lose weight. ”

Obese animals have a greater chance of directly accumulating fat around vital organs if they continue to eat a high-fat diet. From a weight-loss perspective, a little healthy fat is essential, but anything more than that is only going to cause problems.

Premium Protein

When it comes to weight loss, I typically recommend most people start with a high-protein commercial diet. By now you're probably familiar with the Atkins Diet. Dr. Atkins used a high-protein, low-carbohydrate diet to achieve spectacular weight-loss results in humans. A person who strictly adheres to the Atkins Diet will lose weight. The debate over the Atkins Diet in the medical community isn't over whether it works (it does), but over the long-term health repercussions of eating lots of meat, pork, and other high-protein, fatty foods. Does the Atkins approach work for dogs?

Studies in both human and pet nutrition suggested that feeding a high-protein, low-carbohydrate diet could result in weight loss *without reducing calories*. You've seen the headlines, "Eat more and weigh less!" If it sounds too good to be true, it probably is. An April 2003 review published in the *Journal of the American Medical Association* found the number of calories must also be reduced to achieve weight loss, not just changing the nutrient profile. You see, it was too good to be true.

An August 2004 *Journal of Nutrition* study found that dogs fed a high-protein, low-carbohydrate diet lost more weight than dogs fed the same number of calories in a high-carbohydrate diet. While the researchers were unable to determine why the high-protein, low-carbohydrate diet group lost more weight and had a higher lean body mass, they simply concluded it did.

All of the dogs in this study were fed 85 percent of their calculated daily maintenance calories. The high-protein, low-carbohydrate diet contained 52 percent protein, 22 percent carbohydrates and 8 percent fat. The high-carbohydrate control diet contained 28 percent protein, 43 percent carbohydrate, and 11 percent fat.

This study concluded that feeding a high-protein, low-carbohydrate diet offered several advantages over a low-calorie, high-fiber diet. The first advantage was the difficulty in adhering to a severely low-calorie feeding regimen. Most dogs become quite vocal about being fed less, leading their owners to cheat. High-protein diets create greater satiety, leading to less begging. The second reason was that adding fiber to replace calories and create "fullness" caused decreased palatability and increase in stool volume (that's research-speak for "doesn't taste as good and makes the dog poop a lot").

A 2009 study published in the *Veterinary Journal* conducted by researchers at the University of Liverpool also found that a high-protein diet helps promote weight loss in dogs. In this study they added more fiber to the weight-loss diet to see what effect, if any, the added fiber had. The added fiber helped not only for weight loss but satiety in the dogs.

Why Is Protein Important for Weight Loss?

High-protein diets help preserve lean muscle mass. When a dog's body doesn't receive enough calories, as when dieting, it turns to its own tissues to obtain energy. This is how dogs and people lose weight and shrink their waistlines. The body has two basic choices: burn fat or muscle. What really happens is that the body generally digests some of both during weight loss. The goal of weight reduction is to lose fat, not muscle. If a dog is suddenly fed less of a normal maintenance diet, it may consume less protein than it needs. If the amount of food and therefore protein are reduced, the body turns to its own muscles to obtain the missing protein. To combat muscle loss, high-protein diets are used.

How Much Protein Should I Feed My Dog?

For weight loss, I look for a diet containing at least 30 percent protein. More is often better. At the low end, a diet containing close to 25 percent protein may work for your dog if calories remain low. Adding fiber may also result in lower protein and fat content, depending on the formulation. The question with increased fiber is not whether it will help your dog lose weight—it will—but whether it helps maintain muscle mass or causes increased stool. Combining high-protein with high-fiber works well in most cases and is becoming more popular with food producers.

> **For weight loss, I recommend looking for a diet containing at least 30 percent protein—more is often better.**

A high-protein diet strategy is often successful for many dogs. If your dog has certain underlying medical conditions such as liver or kidney disease, though, this approach may not be suitable. Once your dog's ideal weight is reached, I recommend changing to a lower-calorie, normal-protein diet.

Does Feeding a High-Protein Diet Cause Kidney Failure?

A common misconception is that feeding a high-protein diet causes kidney failure in dogs. Fortunately, scientific studies prove this is false. A landmark study published in the June 1986 issue of *Kidney International* examined this very question. In the study, researchers evaluated dogs with only one-quarter (25 percent) of normal kidney tissue remaining. The researchers then fed the dogs a diet containing either 56 percent, 27 percent, or 19 percent protein for four years. The scientists did not find a relationship between death and the amount of protein the dogs were fed. Their results did not support the hypothesis that feeding a high-protein diet had significant adverse effect on renal function in dogs.

Another study, published in the September 2005 issue of *Nutrition and Metabolism,* also concluded that feeding a high-protein diet did not contribute to kidney failure. The authors pointed out that more research was needed in healthy animals to fully understand the role protein has in the development of renal disease.

While it appears that feeding your dog a high-protein diet doesn't cause kidney disease, you should not feed a high-protein diet to a dog with kidney disease. Feeding a high-protein diet, especially one in excess of 40 to 50 percent, may worsen any existing kidney failure. This is one of the primary reasons you should have your pet's blood and urine tested prior to beginning a high-protein weight-loss diet.

Quelling Carbohydrate Confusion

Food companies aren't required to share any information with their consumers about carbohydrate content. And most don't, which presents a greater challenge for pet owners with less active dogs who are trying to watch their pet's carb intake. Even more important, if you have an overweight dog developing insulin sensitivity, knowing the carbohydrate content of your food is vitally important. Most dogs simply don't need as many carbohydrates as we're currently feeding them.

In order to fully evaluate your dog's food, you need to know the number of calories each major nutrient category is supplying, including carbohydrates. To find the amount of carbohydrates in your dog's food, add the percentage amount of each nutrient and subtract it from 100 percent. This is not as accurate as we'd like because fiber is considered a carbohydrate, but it gets you close.

Let's take an example from a dog food label and calculate the amount of carbohydrates the food contains.

Guaranteed Analysis	
Crude Protein (Min)	25.0%
Crude Fat (Min)	10.0%
Crude Fiber (Max)	4.0%
Moisture (Max)	14.0%
Calcium (Ca) (Min)	1.1%

100% − (25% + 10% + 14% + 1.1%) − 63.9% gross carbohydrate content
63.9% gross carbohydrate content − 4% fiber = 59.9% carbohydrate content

This dog food is about 60 percent carbohydrates on an as-fed basis.

You may also see "ash" listed on dog foods instead of calcium or other minerals. Ash and calcium are typically only about 1 percent of the food by weight.

To calculate the amount of carbohydrates in the food on a dry-matter (DM) basis, we subtract from 100 percent the amount of fat, protein, fiber, and minerals on a dry-matter basis.

Nutrient	Percentage of Food As Fed	Percentage on Dry-Matter Basis
Crude protein	25	29
Crude fat	10	11.6
Crude fiber	4	4.7
Calcium	1.1	1.3
Carbohydrates	60	53.4

100% − (29% protein DM + 11.6% fat DM + 4.7% fiber DM + 1.3% Calcium [minerals] DM) = 53.4% carbohydrates on a dry-matter basis

This food contains over 53 percent carbohydrates on a dry-matter basis. For an active adult dog, that may not be excessive. For an indoor, overweight, lap potato, 53.4 percent is too much.

Let's look a little closer at the ingredient list to see if we can determine why there are so many carbohydrates.

Carb Patrol: Finding the Hidden Carbs

INGREDIENTS

Ground yellow corn, chicken by-product meal, corn gluten meal, whole wheat flour, animal fat preserved with mixed-tocopherols (form of Vitamin E), rice flour, beef, soy flour, sugar, sorbitol, tricalcium phosphate, water, salt, phosphoric acid, animal digest, potassium chloride, dicalcium phosphate, sorbic acid (a preservative), L-Lysine monohydrochloride, dried peas, dried carrots, calcium carbonate, calcium propionate (a preservative), choline chloride, added color (Yellow 5, Red 40, Yellow 6, Blue 2), DL-Methionine, Vitamin E supplement, zinc sulfate, ferrous sulfate, Vitamin A supplement, manganese sulfate, niacin, Vitamin B-12 supplement, calcium pantothenate, riboflavin supplement, copper sulfate, biotin, garlic oil, thiamine hydrochloride, pyridoxine hydrochlo-

ride, thiamine mononitrate, folic acid, Vitamin D-3 supplement, menadione sodium bisulfite complex (source of Vitamin K activity), calcium
iodate, sodium selenite.

The first five ingredients tell you all you need to know. Three of the
first five ingredients are carbohydrate sources: ground yellow corn,
corn gluten meal, and whole wheat flour. Of the first ten ingredients,
seven are carbohydrates. That's right, 70 percent of the top ten ingredients are carbohydrates. Of the other three, two are protein sources
(good) and the last is added fat (not good). But something more sinis-
ter lurks on the list: sugar. The ninth and tenth ingredients are sweet-
eners. Following the sugar are the salts. There you have it: the terrible
trifecta of fat, sugar, and salt—not exactly optimal when your dog is
on a diet.

Digestibility: How Is Your Dog Using the Food?

You give your dog a cup of food or a treat. She gobbles it up, wants
more, and eventually defecates. What happens to the food between
pig-out and poop? Understanding the basic digestive physiology of
your dog helps you better manage its health and weight.

The major purpose of the digestive system is to modify ingested
nutrients so that they may be used for energy, maintaining the integrity
of tissues, growth, and reproduction. That sounds pretty simple, especially when you consider the tens of millions of biochemical processes
that are involved. Digestion is one of the most complex systems in the
body. The fact that a dog, cow, or person can ingest a leaf from a plant
and turn it into energy or the building blocks of muscles is still a bit
murky in terms of our understanding, which leads us into disagree-
ments on the best or right way to feed ourselves or our pets. While a
plethora of known facts are available, a great deal remains to be discovered about how to optimize the digestive tract of animals.

To review the digestive process of the dog, imagine the actions involved in cleaning your clothes. The first step in washing clothes is to load the washer with the dirty clothes. This is similar to the actions of a dog eating a meal, swallowing the food, and passing it into the stomach. Next, the clothes are mixed with hot water (stomach acids and digestive enzymes) and vigorously tumbled about (the mechanical action of the stomach's grinding). The detergent is added once the clothes are uniformly mixed (pancreatic enzymes and bile), and dirt and stains are broken down. A second cleaning phase is often necessary to fully clean exceptionally dirty clothes (small intestinal bacteria). The clothes washer then spins and removes the water and debris (large intestine absorbing the remaining water and electrolytes and the colon's bacterial fermentation). Finally, the clean clothes are removed and hung out to dry (descending colon, rectum, and defecation). Just as feces may be thought of as food "wrung out" of its nutrients and moisture, so have the dirty clothes been similarly cleaned.

As you begin to evaluate your dog's food, consider one critical nutrition factor the number crunching doesn't tell you: how well can your dog digest and utilize the nutrients? Just because a dog food has 40 percent protein on a dry-matter basis doesn't necessarily mean your dog can optimally use that protein. One dog may be able to fully digest and use beef protein while another develops inflammatory bowel disease. In general, you want to see as many whole-sourced, unprocessed ingredients as possible. Bear in mind you still may see chemical names you're unfamiliar with on the ingredient list. As long as these are vitamin and mineral supplements instead of artificial flavorings and colorings, your dog should be fine.

> **" As you begin to evaluate your dog's food, there's one critical nutrition factor the number crunching doesn't tell you: how well can your dog digest and utilize the nutrients? "**

You should start by examining how digestible the food ingredients are, especially the protein sources. Keep in mind that the guaranteed analysis is only a start in understanding the quality of the food. Dog owners often rely too heavily on the percentages of nutrients found in the guaranteed analysis and forget about the specific ingredients used in the food. Years ago in a highly publicized study, a large pet food manufacturer made a mock product that had a guaranteed analysis of 10 percent protein, 6.5 percent fat, 2.4 percent fiber, and 78 percent moisture. The twist was that the ingredients used and analyzed were old leather work boots, motor oil, crushed coal, and water! "Guaranteed analysis" can be easily manipulated. All of these ingredients met AAFCO's nutrient requirements yet say nothing about safety or bioavailability. While this example was meant as a joke, in 2007, a toxic compound called melamine was added to dog food to falsely boost the analyzed protein content of the food. This resulted in hundreds, if not thousands, of dogs becoming ill and created the largest pet food recall in history. Therefore, digestibility, ingredients, and safety count as much, if not more, than the guaranteed analysis.

Digestibility is a term used to describe how well the body uses a food. In its most basic usage, high digestibility is linked with low stool volume. Stool or feces is produced when there are metabolic and digestive leftovers, which is why we refer to feces as "waste." Some stool production is healthy; when it is associated with optimal fiber amounts, it helps the body digest nutrients and protects against certain intestinal diseases, including colon cancer. Too much stool production often indicates excessive fiber and other unusable ingredients. Most dogs will have the same number of bowel movements as times they are fed. A dog fed an optimal diet twice a day will typically have two bowel movements per day. A dog fed a poorer-quality or low-digestibility diet has more stool production. A dog fed a high-fiber diet often defecates more frequently.

Stool Volume and Consistency

Stool volume or the amount of feces produced is often directly related to the dry-matter digestibility of the food. In a study published in the fourth edition of *Small Animal Clinical Nutrition,* researchers found that dogs fed foods with even small differences in digestibility produced much more feces. Dogs fed a highly digestible diet of 88.5 percent produced less than half the stool volume of dogs fed a common commercial diet with 80 percent energy digestibility. The researchers studied the effects of digestibility on the stool volume of beagles. They commented that these effects may be even greater (i.e., more wet fecal weight—yuck!) in large-breed dogs.

If your dog's stool is soft and unformed or defecation takes place several times a day, the food you're feeding may have low digestibility. High-fiber diets often produce several hard and dry stools a day, although some dogs experience diarrhea or soft stools. Dogs fed a high-fat diet often have soft, runny, and light brown stools, although the color may vary. In addition, high-fat foods are often associated with a strong odor. High-carbohydrate diets can also lead to poorly formed, soft stools.

Ideally, choose a dog food with the protein source you desire and your dog enjoys, a nutrient profile that meets your dog's needs (i.e., a high-protein, low-fat, or high-fiber approach for weight loss), and that produces a normal stool once or twice a day (more if a high-fiber diet is used). This real-world digestibility experiment can be performed each time you see your dog defecate. Mushy, gloppy, poorly formed, stinky feces probably means the diet is less than optimal. Small, firm, well-formed stools that are easy to pick up once or twice a day means you're on the right dietary track.

Nine Signs a Dog Food Isn't Right for Your Dog

1 Diarrhea or constipation. Either one often indicates a digestibility problem in an otherwise healthy dog.

2 Chronic loose, runny, or "melted ice cream" stools. This type of stool even once a day signals that something is wrong. Normal feces should be somewhat firm, well-formed, and a consistent color.

3 Stinky poop. Feces with a strong odor usually results from poorly digested nutrients or excessive fat.

4 Frequent defecation. A dog that needs to defecate four or more times a day may have a problem with the current diet.

5 Dull, flaky, or greasy coat. There may be an issue with a fat source (too much or too little).

6 Smelly dog. A strong doggy odor is often the result of a poor diet.

7 Frequent infections. Frequent ear, skin, or urinary tract infections often indicate a poor diet.

8 Tiredness. Dogs with low energy are probably eating an unhealthy diet.

9 Moodiness. Dogs fed high-sugar treats often experience sugar highs and sugar crashes that may be interpreted as mood swings. Dogs that don't receive adequate omega-3 fatty acids also may undergo behavioral changes.

With some effort and continued diligence, you can feel good feeding your dog a commercial dog food that will help her shed weight. But for any budding gourmets, the next chapter will give guidelines for healthy home-cooked meals.

8

Rx 5: Make Home Cooking Healthy

With our busy lifestyles and many of us eating on the run, we humans rarely eat together anymore. However, feeding your dog healthy, wholesome meals made from scratch is actually easier than you might think. If you can manage it, I recommend the Hybrid Menu for most of my clients.

How the Hybrid Menu Works

The hybrid menu works well for most dog owners and provides a nutritional boost over feeding only a commercial dog food. A hybrid menu means that you prepare your dog's meals two to three times a week. By rotating fresh, whole foods with commercially prepared diets, dogs enjoy maximum nutrition with minimum effort. This hybrid diet also ensures that your dog won't suffer from nutritional deficits often created by feeding only a home-cooked diet.

On days when you prepare your dog's meal, I recommend a high-quality protein source such as wild-caught salmon or hormone-free, free-range chicken or turkey. Combine this protein with a high-quality grain such as quinoa, millet, or brown rice. Add superfoods such as sweet potatoes, kale, spinach, kelp, and broccoli to keep a healthy dog healthier. In essence, you feed your dog what you should be eating every day!

These meals are quick and easy to prepare and most can be made in advance and stored in the refrigerator or frozen until you use them. Of course, the key to weight loss is sticking to the recommended number of calories, which can make calculating home-made meals somewhat challenging. Most of my weight-loss recipes, which you'll find at the end of this chapter, contain less than 200 calories per cup. Because they are highly palatable, you may see your dog gulp them down and want more. Don't give in to the urge to splurge. Just because your dog really likes his diet food doesn't mean you should give him more.

Hybrid Menu Tips

Alternate. By alternating food sources every two to four days you maximize nutrition with minimal effort.

Rotate. Rotating your protein, vegetable, and carb sources monthly will help optimize your pet's natural metabolism.

Portion control. Your dog will likely *love* the home-prepared meals, but don't forget that weight loss is the goal.

Protein power. One of my main reasons for using the hybrid diet is the chance to boost protein. When in doubt, offer more fish and meat (watching the calories, of course).

Favorite fishes. My personal preference is to use fish protein sources as often as possible. Salmon, albacore tuna, bluefish, sardines, and other oily fishes are ideal. Avoid farm-raised fish, and select wild and freshly caught when available.

Act locally. Feed fresh, in-season, and locally grown ingredients whenever possible.

Add kelp. Kelp is a great source of sodium, calcium, vitamin A, folic acid, iodine, and other minerals. Some researchers even claim it helps with weight loss. One half to 1 teaspoon daily is adequate for dogs being fed 100% home-prepared meals; use kelp less frequently for dogs eating some commercial food.

Stock up on sweet potatoes. Sweet potatoes are one of my favorite vegetables for dogs. They are rich in dietary fiber, naturally occurring sugars, complex carbohydrates, protein, vitamins A and C, iron, and calcium. I recommend feeding your dog sweet potatoes at least weekly.

Beet it. Beets are a good source of dietary fiber and contain powerful nutrients, including folate, manganese and potassium, vitamin C, magnesium, iron, copper, and phosphorus. Try them raw (watch out, the juice stains), grated, cooked, or (my favorite) juiced beets.

Mince it up. If your dog doesn't like a vegetable, it may be the texture, not the taste. When adding veggies to the diet, try mincing, pureeing, or finely chopping them before adding them to your dog's food.

Try hot and cold. Some dogs like their food slightly warm while others seem to prefer it a little cool. If your dog doesn't eat your prepared meal, try changing the temperature. If you warm it in the microwave, be sure to test the temperature of the food with your finger before serving.

Ketchup. Just like kids, dogs seem to eat more foods when covered in ketchup. Preferably choose one with no corn syrup. One teaspoon has about 10 calories so be stingy with your picky eater.

Dump carbs, add veggies. A convenient way to add fresh foods to your dog's diet is to substitute treats and biscuits with vegetables. Baby carrots, sliced cucumbers, sugar snap peas, celery, asparagus, and broccoli are all packed with phytonutrients to keep your dog healthy.

Fish oil. Fish oil added to the food not only improves nutritional value, but also enhances palatability. Be sure to try fish oils formulated for dogs, which taste better to them (e.g., Nutramax Welactin, Nordic Naturals Pet Cod Liver Oil).

Double time. Even the busiest pet parent can find time to prepare a simple, nutritious meal for their dog twice a week. Making one of my weight-loss meals takes only a few minutes.

Freeze frame. Many healthy dog meals can be refrigerated or frozen. Cooking in bulk can also save you time and money. Whenever possible, use freshly prepared ingredients, but when time runs short, thaw it out!

Canine Cooking 101

Some people love to spend time in their kitchens. If you like to cook and you're able to make homemade meals for your dog, there are some important guidelines you need to follow to ensure his nutrient needs are being met.

Protein Source

The most important part of your dog's diet is the protein source. I strongly recommend you vary the protein and carbohydrate sources weekly in home prepared meals and every two to three months if you feed a commercial diet. In the rare cases of reported nutritional deficiencies of dogs fed homemade diets, the cause is typically feeding a strict set of ingredients with little, if any, variation. Ideally, you'll use a protein source without added antibiotics and hormones and raised in a humane and sustainable environment. While I believe these conditions create more nutritious foods, the real reason you should choose humane and organic sources is for the health of our planet and future generations. For these reasons, my top two protein sources are farm-raised turkey and wild-caught salmon. Both are readily available and relatively inexpensive. If you prefer to feed other meats, lean cuts of beef, pork, and chicken are recommended.

- Homemade meals should have a final protein content of 30 percent to 50 percent for weight loss—typically one part meat for every one to two parts carbohydrate or grain. For a maintenance diet, the ratio should be 25-30% protein and 75-70%, vegetable, carbohydrate, or grain.
- If you're using a high-quality protein source, the amino acid profile should be adequate for your dog. Adding liver or egg occasionally can make up for any potential deficiencies.
- If you are feeding a nonmeat or vegetarian diet to your dog, add 200 mg to 500 mg of taurine daily. Your veterinarian can test

your dog's taurine levels to ensure that adequate amounts are present in your dog's diet.

• Eggs, soybeans, pinto beans, and chickpeas are excellent sources of nonmeat dietary protein. Dogs sometimes have difficulty digesting beans, so make sure you are closely monitoring weight, coat appearance, stools, and overall health status.

Carbohydrates

Carbohydrates or grains are your dog's preferred source of energy. Prime sources include cooked corn, rice, wheat, potato, barley, quinoa (also rich in protein), couscous, tapioca, brown rice, millet, sweet potato, and oatmeal. We don't know the digestibility of the wide variety of carbohydrates available to us. A simple way to tell if your dog seems able to digest a given homemade diet is the poop test. If your dog's stools become more voluminous, runny, or loose, or if your dog becomes constipated, alter your ingredients or amounts. This is only a crude indicator, but a dog with runny or abnormally large or numerous stools probably is experiencing digestive disorders.

Fat

For weight loss, you probably don't need to add fat to your dog's diet. I do, however, recommend supplementing omega-3 fatty acids (DHA/EPA) in your dog's diet. Even if you're feeding a salmon- or sardine-based diet, I recommend that you add fish oils to your dog's diet daily. If you find that, despite adding fish oils, your dog's coat appears dull or lusterless, you may want to try feeding sirloin or chuck cuts that contain more fat than lean trimmings.

Calcium

Because most homemade recipes contain more protein than commercial diets, you'll need to supplement calcium in your dog's diet because meats contain more phosphorus and little calcium. If your dog doesn't ingest additional calcium, the ratio between phosphorus and calcium can become unbalanced. Adding about 1 g of calcium carbonate per 15 pounds daily (thus, a 30-pound dog would receive 2 g per day and a 7½-pound dog would need 0.5 g daily) should be adequate for most dogs. I do not recommend feeding bone meal or calcium phosphorus. Because bone contains phosphorus, these additives may not help balance the calcium-to-phosphorus ratio appropriately.

Vitamins and Trace Minerals

In a perfect world, you and your dog could receive everything needed nutritionally from what you ate. Due to a variety of factors—nutrient-depleted soils, modern farming and food processing procedures, and limited fruit and vegetable consumption, to name but a few—we can't depend on what we eat to provide us with optimal levels of vitamins and minerals. For this reason, I strongly recommend the addition of supplements to fill any potential dietary gaps (see supplements, Chapter 12). The easiest way to give your dog these nutrients is by adding a pre-mix. Currently the best and safest source is Balance IT (www.balanceit.com). On their website you can create homemade recipes and purchase vitamin and mineral supplements. In addition, if you use salt in your dog's food, be sure to occasionally use iodized salt. Sea salt does not contain iodine, an essential nutrient in dogs. If you feed a home-cooked diet or if you feel more comfortable giving your dog additional vitamins, be sure to avoid giving excessive amounts of the fat-soluble vitamins A, D, E, and K.

People Foods to Avoid Feeding Your Dog

If you're going to feed your dog healthy human foods from time to time, you should know to avoid certain foods. Some of these items are obvious no-no's while others may surprise you. Some are safe in small amounts; others are deadly even in tiny doses. This list is certainly far from comprehensive and is based on the National Animal Poison Control Center's recommendations (www.aspca.org/apcc).

Foods Known to Be Toxic

Chocolate, Coffee, and Caffeinated Products. The three Cs contain a class of substances known as methylxanthines. In dogs, these compounds can cause vomiting and diarrhea, panting, increased thirst and urination, hyperactivity, abnormal heartbeats, tremors, and seizures and can even lead to death in certain circumstances. Dark and baking chocolates have the greatest toxicity, while milk chocolate has a relatively low toxicity level.

Alcohol. Each year around the holidays, scores of dogs are poisoned when they counter-surf their way into leftover cocktails and beer. Dogs are very sensitive to the effects of alcohol and can become toxic quickly. Vomiting, diarrhea, depression, difficulty breathing, tremors, abnormal blood acidity, coma, and even death can result from alcohol ingestion in dogs. Never give your dog alcohol or food containing alcohol.

Avocado. Avocados contain an ingredient that causes vomiting and diarrhea in dogs.

Macadamia Nuts. Macadamia nuts are popular ingredients used in many desserts, and we all know how our dogs love cookies. Unfortunately, chemicals in macadamia nuts can potentially cause weakness, depression, vomiting, tremors, and high temperatures in dogs.

Grapes and Raisins. There have been a few cases of grapes and raisins causing kidney problems in dogs. To date, the cause of kidney toxicity has not been determined nor has a toxic dosage been established. For this reason, I do not recommend feeding your dog raisins, grapes, or grape juice.

Onions, Garlic, and Chives. There have been several high-profile cases of concerns over pet food recipes containing garlic. The fact is that these ingredients pose more of a potential risk to cats than dogs. If a dog consumes a large amount of onions, garlic, or chives at one sitting, toxicity, including life-threatening anemia, may develop. Otherwise, occasionally feeding your dog small amounts will not likely cause any problems.

Xylitol. Xylitol is a popular sweetener used in many foods such as gum, candy, and baked goods. In dogs, it has been associated with liver failure. Avoid feeding your dog any food containing Xylitol.

Raw or Undercooked Meat, Eggs, and Bones. Raw or undercooked meat and eggs can contain bacteria such as *Salmonella* and *E. coli* that can be harmful to both people and pets. Raw eggs also contain an enzyme, avidin, which decreases the absorption of the B vitamin biotin. Dogs that consume raw eggs frequently may develop skin and coat problems.

People seem to want to give their dogs bones. Feeding bones can be very dangerous because your dog might choke or tear its intestinal tract as bone splinters pass through it. Say no to bones.

Green Parts of Potatoes and Tomatoes. Feeding your dog potatoes and tomatoes is safe; just avoid the leaves, stems, and any other green parts. If you were to feed your dog large quantities of these vegetables raw, your dog could become sick, so add them to recipes in moderate amounts. Cooking them definitely reduces any potential toxicity.

Rhubarb Leaves. Rhubarb leaves may contain high levels of calcium oxalates that can cause kidney damage. Skip the rhubarb pie for your dogs (they'll thank you).

Myth Makers

These foods are sometimes reported as harmful when there's no evidence to support this claim. Of course, any of these foods can cause potential problems if fed too much or to an unhealthy or sensitive dog.

Acai

Almonds

Anise oil

Apples (except the stems and leaves, which can be toxic in large amounts)

Brazil nuts

Cantaloupe

Carob

Coconut oil and milk

Coriander

Corn

Cranberries and cranberry juice

Cucumbers

Mushrooms

Oranges

Parsley

Peanuts

Pistachios

Pomegranate

Shrimp (cooked)

Sorbitol (as used in dog toothpastes)

Spinach (don't feed to dogs with kidney disease or certain types of bladder stones)

Watermelon

Yogurt

Zucchini

Other Food Risks

Among the other risks that owners should consider when planning a diet for their dogs are allergies and raw foods. Each can present certain problems in individual cases.

Food Allergies

Some dogs are born with a genetic predisposition toward developing certain allergies, including toward foods. If you compare recent studies on food allergies in dogs, you find these are the most common offending ingredients:

Beef

Chicken

Dairy

Egg

Fish

Lamb/mutton

Pork

Rabbit

Soy

Wheat

The most current scientific studies do not support the belief that grains cause the majority of food allergies in dogs.

Raw Has Risks

Feeding your dog a raw-food diet is appealing on many levels. Proponents argue that this is how dogs evolved, and by feeding raw, uncooked meat you're simply doing what nature intended. Further, advocates argue that processing and cooking food destroys valuable micronutrients. They claim that by feeding raw foods you're simply preserving these healthy ingredients.

I agree that processed foods should be avoided as much as is practicable. Excessive rendering and heat extrusion can indeed sometimes alter proteins and nutrients. The extent of this damage is related to the specific process involved.

In a perfect world, none of the food we or our pets eat would be commercially processed. However, we don't live in that world, so we must make our decisions based on reality.

As for the myth that cooking methods destroy nutrients, there is evidence that heating may favorably alter certain foods. A June 2005 study published in *Food Chemistry* found that cooking legumes significantly enhanced the absorption of protein and carbohydrates. Another fascinating study, conducted by faculty from Harvard University, added more fuel to the cooking fire. In the September 2003 issue of *Comparative Biochemistry and Physiology*, scientists reported that humans eating a purely raw-food diet had low energy levels and impaired reproductive function. They suggested that because humans have cooked for at least tens, if not hundreds, of thousands of years, our physiology had adapted to cooked foods. Because dogs evolved alongside humans, it's not a stretch to postulate they may have experienced similar changes. No human foragers have ever been shown to live without cooking. These studies bring into serious question the whole "we evolved from eating raw meat" theory. That's not to say there aren't health benefits to eating fresh, unprocessed foods. There certainly are; however, I am greatly concerned about feeding a dog or person uncooked meat.

There are currently three major raw-diet approaches. The first recommends commercially available dog foods that use raw foods as their ingredients. The second strategy employs use of a commercially produced grain and supplement mix into which you add raw meats. The third option is a complete home-prepared raw-food diet commonly referred to as a BARF (bones and raw food) diet.

All three approaches have been shown to have contamination problems. A popular raw-food diet company, Evanger's, had its operating permit suspended in June 2009. According to the FDA, Evanger's deviated from safe food production protocols. The FDA stated these deviations "could result in under-processed pet foods, which can allow the survival and growth of *Clostridium botulinum (C. botulinum)*, a bacterium that causes botulism in some animals as well as in humans." The FDA cannot stop Evanger's from making its raw foods, but the FDA can prevent the company from selling them outside its home state of Illinois.

The biggest issue with raw foods involves bacterial contamination, which can cause disease in both pets and people. In November 2006, the Canadian Veterinary Medical Association and the Public Health Agency of Canada issued a warning: "There is evidence of potential health risks for pets fed raw meat based diets, and for humans in contact with such pets." The most common route of infection is through direct contact with the raw meat or feces. In a household with young children, the fact is that an apparently healthy dog could be transmitting pathogenic bacteria such as *Salmonella* or *E. coli* through the feces. Children could accidentally step in or touch feces and eventually contract illness.

EYE ON THE SCIENCE

The Risks of Raw

One study published in June 2002 in the *Canadian Veterinary Journal* evaluated salmonella contamination in dogs fed a BARF diet with raw chicken. *Salmonella* was isolated from 80 percent of the BARF diets and 30 percent of the stools of dogs fed a BARF diet. The researchers issued a stern warning against feeding dogs raw chicken, especially in families with young children, older adults, and family members who may be ill or immune-compromised.

A study published in the February 15, 2006, *Journal of the American Veterinary Medical Association* investigated bacterial contamination of commercially prepared raw-food diets. They evaluated 240 samples from twenty raw-meat diets for dogs (containing beef, lamb, chicken, or turkey) over a period of one year. To compare as control samples, twenty-four samples from two normal adult commercial dry dog foods and twenty-four samples from two canned dog foods were used. Of the raw foods, 59.6 percent were found contaminated with *E. coli*, and 7.1 percent contained *Salmonella*. Ten of the twenty-one (47.6 percent) raw-meat diets contained *E. coli* during each of the four sampling periods.

These studies were published long before the pet food recall of 2007 and served as an early warning to what has become a serious health threat to both dogs and humans.

In addition to raw meats, handling raw eggs, bones, pig ears, and raw food treats also presents the risk of humans contracting an infectious disease. Because of these concerns and the fact that feeding raw meats has not been proven to confer any additional health benefits (only the risk of disease), the FDA does not recommend feeding your dog raw meats. I strongly concur with that opinion. Raw can be dangerous—except when we're talking about many vegetables, although you should always wash them first.

Treats: Trash 'Em or Trade 'Em

Ah, treats. Everyone enjoys giving treats to their dogs. A treat for going outside and going to potty in the morning, repeated at lunch and in the evening. A treat just before you go to work and again when you return to reward good behavior. An after-dinner goody because your dog begged during the meal but didn't bark.

But who are the treats *really* for? They're mainly for us. They absolve us of the guilt we feel when we leave or because we don't have thirty minutes to walk them or the fact that we can't give them a piece of our apple pie (at least not a large one).

Dog treats are more for people than dogs, which is why they're made in shapes, sizes, and colors that are familiar to people. "Sausage," "beef," "real meat," and other dog-tasty terms are used. Dogs don't care about names, shapes, sizes, or colors.

The trouble with treats is that they're full of sugar, fat, and salt. They're carb-grenades destroying your dog's health one tasty morsel at a time. While the package may describe a healthy high-protein snack, the ingredients reveal another story. As you've already learned, high-sugar foods create a response similar to cocaine in your dog's brain. Your and your dog's willpower are simply no match for these deep neurochemical responses. It's in a dog's basic physiology to crave calorically dense foods such as those containing large quantities of sugar and fat.

Throw out any commercial treats, unless they are low-calorie (less than 15 calories) and low in fat (less than 10 percent). Get rid of them. Now. You and your dog don't have enough discipline to avoid reaching for a tasty morsel when things get rough.

I recently had a client who finally took me up on helping her obese dachshund lose weight. Her dog was beginning to experience back and knee problems, and blood tests detected insulin resistance. We developed a feeding and exercise plan, and everything seemed to be going well . . . until she dropped this atom bomb: "Dr. Ward, this all sounds great. Trouble is, I just bought a 40-pound bag of the old dog food. I'll get started as soon as I finish my new bag. Besides, we've still got loads of dog bones I need to go through before I stop giving goodies."

A 40-pound bag of food for a dachshund? Boxes of treats? We're talking a minimum three months before her dog finishes that. I never advocate wasting; plenty of animal shelters could benefit from a donation of food and treats.

The best advice is to trash your treats unless they are low in calories or swap them with some healthy alternatives (see below). There's simply no room for those empty calories and brain-altering chemicals in your dog's new healthier lifestyle.

Treats That Fill Up, Not Out

Baby carrots	2–3 calories per carrot
Stringless sugar snap peas	2 calories per pea
Cucumber	1 calorie per ¼" slice
Apple	16 calories per slice (⅛) large red apple
Asparagus	3–5 calories per spear
Celery	6 calories per 7–8" stalk
Broccoli	5–6 calories per floret
Banana	7–9 calories per ½" slice
Blueberries	31 calories per ½ cup
Strawberries	23 calories per ½ cup (whole)
Watermelon	23 calories per ½ cup (diced)
Pumpkin	21 calories per ½ cup (canned, without salt)
Sweet potato	58 calories in ½ medium sweet potato (without skin, cooked or boiled)
Nonfat Plain Yogurt	64 calories per 4 ounces (½ cup)

As you can see, how much and what we feed our dogs is the major factor when it comes to their weight. However, another critical component of losing weight and improving health is exercise. In addition to the healthy recipes that follow, the next chapter will give you ideas, advice, and suggested activities to get your dog her fittest.

You'll notice the recipes include nutritional information for each ingredient. By knowing this, you can customize each recipe for your dog. Individual ingredient information is not included in the treats because they are low in calories and contain a minimal number of ingredients. Bon appétit!

Oh-Mega Salmon

Makes 6 cups

	Calories	Protein (g)	Fat (g)	Carbs (g)	Fiber (g)
1 14½-ounce can or 3½ cups cooked salmon	1,143	162.6	50.2	0	4
1 cup chopped kale	34	2.2	.5	6.7	1.3
½ cup chopped green beans	17	.1	.1	4	2
1 cup cooked quinoa	226	9	3.9	46.92	4
1 Tbsp kelp powder	2	.1	.1	.5	.1
Totals 6 cups	*1,422*	*174*	*54.8*	*58.5*	*7.4*
Per Cup	*237*	*29*	*9.1*	*9.8*	*1.2*

- Place the kale and green beans in a blender or food processor and blend until minced or pureed.

- In a bowl, combine the vegetable mixture, salmon, quinoa, and kelp powder and mix thoroughly. Divide into portions appropriate for your pet's caloric intake.

Kitchen Hints & Tips

✓ Kale, spinach, and broccoli should be avoided in dogs with kidney disease or certain types of bladder stones.

✓ Quinoa (pronounced KEEN-wa), referred to as the mother of all grains, is a highly nutritious seed, and a good source of fiber and protein. It's also easy to digest.

TURKEY PIE

Makes 6½ cups

	Calories	Protein (g)	Fat (g)	Carbs (g)	Fiber (g)
3½ cups cooked chopped turkey (*white meat*)	686	147.9	5.9	0	0
1 cup chopped raw broccoli	31	2.6	.4	6	2.4
½ cup chopped apples	33	0	.1	8.6	1.5
1½ cups cooked millet	311	9.2	2.6	61.9.	3.4
1 Tbsp kelp powder	2	.1	.1	.5	.1
Totals 6½ cups	*1063*	*159.8*	*9.1*	*77*	*7.4*
Per cup	*163.5*	*24.5*	*1.4*	*11.8*	*1.1*

- Rinse the turkey breast with cold water and pat dry. Wrap the breast with aluminum foil, folding the edges to seal in moisture. Place in a baking pan. Roast at 350°F for 20 minutes per pound. Open the aluminum foil, being careful not to burn yourself on the escaping steam. Chop once cooled.
- Combine the broccoli and apples in a blender or food processor and blend until minced or pureed.
- In a bowl, combine the vegetable mixture with the turkey, millet, and kelp powder and mix thoroughly. Divide into portions appropriate for your pet's caloric intake.

Kitchen Hints & Tips

✓ Fresh fruits and vegetables are healthiest but if you need to save time use frozen foods, not canned.

✓ If your dog doesn't like raw veggies, try lightly steaming them instead.

✓ Millet is a nutritious and low-allergen grain.

Eggs-Cellently Delicious Eggs

Makes approximately 5½ cups

	Calories	Protein (g)	Fat (g)	Carbs (g)	Fiber (g)
½ cup chopped celery	7	.3	.1	1.7	.8
½ cup chopped carrots	26	.6	.1	6.1	1.8
½ cup chopped spinach	3	.4	.1	.5	.3
2 cups chopped boiled eggs (*about 5 eggs*)	390	34	63.2	0	0
2 cups 2% cottage cheese	407	62.1	8.6	16.3	0
1 Tbsp kelp powder	2	.1	.1	.5	.1
2 Tbsps nutritional yeast	45	8	.5	5	4
Total 5½ cups	*880*	*105.5*	*72.7*	*30.1*	*7*
Per cup	*160*	*19.2*	*13.2*	*5.5*	*1.3*

- Place the vegetables in a blender or food processor and blend until minced or pureed, whichever your dog prefers.
- In a bowl, combine the vegetable mixture with the eggs, cottage cheese, and kelp powder, and mix thoroughly. Divide into portions appropriate for your pet's caloric intake.

Kitchen
Hints
& Tips

✓ Kelp is a sea vegetable and has a salty taste. It has a high content of natural plant iodine, is highly nutritious, and is considered a superfood for dogs. Kelp is reported to improve energy and enhance the immune system.

✓ Nutritional yeast is a non-active form of yeast that has a delicious nutty, cheesy flavor. It is not to be confused with brewer's yeast. Nutritional yeast contains 18 amino acids and 15 different minerals and is an added source of protein.

B Lean Steak

Makes 5½ cups

	Calories	Protein (g)	Fat (g)	Carbs (g)	Fiber (g)
2 cups cooked chopped lean sirloin steak	959	154.5	33.7	0	0
1 cup cooked barley	193	3.5	.6	44.3	6
1 cup chopped sugar snap peas	124	8.2	.2	7.4	2.5
½ chopped carrot	26	.6	.1	6.1	1.8
1 cup chopped raw kale	34	2.2	.5	6.7	1.3
1 Tbsp kelp powder	2	.1	.1	.5	.1
Total 5½ cups	*1338*	*169.1*	*35.2*	*65*	*11.7*
Per cup	*243*	*30.8*	*6.4*	*11.8*	*2.1*

- In a nonstick skillet, place cubed lean steak and cook over medium heat until cooked thoroughly. Chop the steak once cooled.
- Combine the peas, carrots, and kale in a blender or food processor and blend until minced or pureed.
- In a bowl, combine the vegetable mixture with the steak, barley, and kelp powder and mix thoroughly. Divide into portions appropriate for your pet's caloric intake.

Kitchen Hints & Tips

✓ Kale needs to be chopped or chewed to release the sulfur-containing phytonutrients that make this one of nature's superfoods.

The frozen vegetables you purchase at the supermarket are blanched prior to freezing to prevent them from turning brown during freezing and stop vitamin loss. Fresh vegetables stored in the refrigerator or pantry for more than three days have lost enough of their vitamins and minerals to make frozen vegetables more nutritious.

CHICKEN AND RICE

Makes 5 cups

	Calories	Protein (g)	Fat (g)	Carbs (g)	Fiber (g)
2½ cups chopped cooked chicken breast	578	108.6	12.6	0	0
1 cup sweet potato (*medium sweet potato*)	180	4	.4	41.4	1.8
½ cup cooked brown rice	108	2.5	.9	22.4	6.6
½ cup chopped spinach	3.5	.4	.1	.5	.3
½ cup chopped celery	7	<.1	.1	1.7	.8
1 Tbsp kelp powder	2	.1	.1	.5	.1
Total 5 cups	*878.5*	*115.7*	*14.2*	*66.5*	*9.6*
Per cup	*176*	*23*	*2.8*	*13.3*	*1.9*

- In a nonstick skillet, place cubed chicken and cook over medium high heat approximately 8 to 10 minutes, until cooked thoroughly. Chop or dice the chicken once cooled.
- Wrap an unpeeled sweet potato in a wet paper towel (prick with a fork in a few places first). Microwave for 10 to 12 minutes.
- Combine the spinach and celery in a blender or food processor and blend until minced or pureed.
- In a bowl, combine the vegetable mixture with the chicken, sweet potato, brown rice, and kelp powder and mix thoroughly. Divide into portions appropriate for your pet's caloric intake.

SOY GOOD VEGGIE MIX

Makes 6 cups

	Calories	Protein (g)	Fat (g)	Carbs (g)	Fiber (g)
3½ cups tofu (*28 ounces*)	1151	125.3	69.1	34.1	18.3
½ cup cooked quinoa	113	4.5	2	23.5	2
½ cup chopped zucchini	10	.8	.1	2.1	.7
½ cup chopped kale	17	1.1	.3	3.4	.7
1 cup chopped carrots	52	1.2	.2	12.2	3.6
1 Tbsp kelp powder	2	.1	.1	.5	.1
¼ cup nutritional yeast	45	6	.5	5	3
Total 6 cups	*1390*	*141*	*72.3*	*80.8*	*29.4*
Per cup	*231.6*	*23.5*	*12*	*13.5*	*4.9*

- In a nonstick skillet, crumble the tofu and add ¼ cup of nutritional yeast. Heat for 5 minutes over low heat to blend the flavors.
- Combine the zucchini, kale, and carrots in a blender or food processor and blend until minced or pureed.
- In a bowl, combine the vegetable mixture with the tofu, quinoa, and kelp powder and mix thoroughly. Divide into portions appropriate for your pet's caloric intake.

Kitchen Hints & Tips

✓ Be sure to rinse the quinoa prior to cooking to remove the bitter saponin coating which is believed to be a natural insect repellant.

✓ ¼ cup cooked quinoa yields approximately 1 cup of cooked quinoa.

✓ Stay away from processed soy and stick with tofu or soybeans for a healthier meal.

✓ Many vegetables have been associated with reducing the risk of cancer. In addition to fighting cancer, vegetables help regulate blood sugar, boost the immune system and aid in weight loss.

Chum and Get It Fish

Makes 3 cups

	Calories	Protein (g)	Fat (g)	Carbs (g)	Fiber (g)
2 3.75-ounce cans of sardines packed in water	340	36.9	19.8	0	0
½ cup chopped celery	7	<.1	.1	1.7	.8
½ chopped carrot	26	.6	.1	6.1	1.8
½ cup blueberries	41	1.1	.4	21	3.5
½ cup lowfat (2%) cottage cheese	102	15.5	2.1	4.1	0
2 Tbsps parsley	2	.2	.1	.5	.3
Total 3 cups	560	54.4	22.6	33.4	6.4
Per cup	187	18	7.5	11	2

- Combine the celery and carrots in a blender or food processor and blend until minced or pureed.
- In a bowl, combine the sardines, vegetable mixture, blueberries, cottage cheese, and parsley and mix thoroughly. Divide into portions appropriate for your pet's caloric intake.

Kitchen Hints & Tips

✓ Sardines are nutritional powerhouses: In addition to CoQ10, they are a great source of vitamin B12, selenium, omega-3 oils, protein, phosphorus, and vitamin D.

EDAMAME

Makes 5½ cups

	Calories	Protein (g)	Fat (g)	Carbs (g)	Fiber (g)
3½ cups cooked and shelled edamame beans	888	77.8	40.3	69.9	26.5
½ cup cooked quinoa	113	4.5	2	23.5	2
½ cup chopped broccoli	15	1.3	.2	3	1.2
½ cup chopped kale	17	1.1	.3	3.4	.7
½ chopped carrot	26	.6	.1	6.1	1.8
1 Tbsp kelp powder	2	.1	.1	.5	.1
¼ cup nutritional yeast	45	6	.5	5	3
Total 5½ cups	*1106*	*93.4*	*43.5*	*111.4*	*36.3*
Per cup	*201*	*17.0*	*12*	*20.3*	*6.6*

- In a medium saucepan, put 5 to 6 cups of water and bring to a boil over medium-high heat. Add 3½ cups raw edamame beans and boil for 3 to 4 minutes. Drain well.
- Combine the broccoli, kale, and carrots in a blender or food processor and blend until minced or pureed.
- In a bowl, combine the vegetable mixture with the edamame beans, quinoa, kelp powder, and nutritional yeast and mix thoroughly. Divide into portions appropriate for your pet's caloric intake.

Kitchen Hints & Tips

✓ Soy is a good source of protein for dogs and is hypoallergenic.

✓ Quinoa is a gluten-free, high-fiber source of complete protein.

Sweet Potato Cookies

Makes 4 dozen

1 large cooked sweet potato	162
1 banana	107
½ Tbsp vegetable oil	62
½ cup quinoa flour	360

• Preheat oven to 350°F.
• In a medium bowl, mix the sweet potato and banana until well blended.
• Add the vegetable oil.
• Mix the quinoa flour with the wet ingredients.
• Place 1 teaspoon of the dough on a nonstick baking sheet and lightly flatten.
• Bake for 30 minutes

Calories per Treat: 14 to 15

QUICHE BITES

Makes 16

½ cup minced vegetables (*celery, carrots, zucchini, spinach*)

2 medium eggs

Pinch of kelp

- Preheat oven to 350°F. Generously coat a non-stick miniature muffin pan with non-stick cooking spray.
- In a bowl, whisk eggs. Add vegetables and kelp and blend.
- Evenly distribute the mixture into the mini-muffin pan.
- Bake for 10 to 12 minutes.

Calories per Treat: 11

SALMON ROLL-OVERS

Makes 18

1 7-ounce can of salmon

⅓ cup of oat flour

1 Tbsp of minced parsley

• Preheat oven to 350°F. Spray a non-stick miniature baking sheet.
• In a medium-sized bowl, mix all of the ingredients until well blended.
• Roll the mixture into 1-inch balls and place on non-stick cooking sheet.
• Bake for 12 to 15 minutes.

Calories per Treat: 23

Kitchen
Hints
& Tips

✓ If you don't have oat flour, just blend dry oats in a food processor. You can also substitute other healthy flours, such as quinoa or amaranth.

Yogurt Pops

Makes 15

1 small ripe banana

1 cup plain, non-fat yogurt

- Blend the banana with the yogurt.
- Pour into a 15-count ice cube tray and place in the freezer.
- When frozen, remove from the tray and serve one at a time.

Calories per Pop: 15

Kitchen Hints & Tips

✓ Yogurt is good for digestive health in dogs as well as people. Yogurt that contains live bacterial cultures can fortify with immune system. Choose only unsweetened yogurts.

Turkey Meatballs

Makes 30

6 ounces lean ground turkey

½ cup chopped carrots

½ cup ground quinoa or oatmeal

Pinch of kelp

- Preheat oven to 400°F.
- Place beef and carrots in a food processor and blend until smooth.
- Add remaining ingredients and blend until mixed.
- Roll into 1-inch balls and place on a non-stick cooking sheet.
- Bake for 15 minutes.

Calories per Meatball: 17

EARTH BISCUITS

Makes 72 cookies

2 cups garbanzo bean flour

1½ teaspoons baking powder

½ cup chopped carrot

¼ cup thawed frozen peas

½ cup packed spinach

2 Tbsps tomato paste

½ teaspoon tumeric

1 teaspoon basil

1 teaspoon oregano

⅛ to ¼ cup water

- Preheat the oven to 350°F.
- Place the carrots, peas, spinach, garlic, tomato paste, and water in a food processor and puree.
- Add the flour, baking powder, basil, and oregano and pulse until blended. Spray an 8 x 10-inch pan with non-stick coating then lightly coat with flour.
- Spread the dough into the pan and score into 56 square pieces. Bake for 30 minutes. Remove from the oven and let cool.

Calories per Cookie: 11

 Kitchen Hints & Tips

✓ Garbanzo flour is made from grinding chick peas and is an excellent source of protein.

✓ Tumeric is a popular spice in South Asian and Middle Eastern cooking. It is believed to have anti-inflammatory and healing properties.

Blueberry Mutt-ins

Makes 36 muffins

½ cup quinoa flour

½ cup oat flour

½ teaspoon cinnamon

½ teaspoon baking soda

¾ cup fresh or thawed blueberries

1 cup applesauce

1 egg

¼ cup water

- Preheat oven to 350°F.
- Combine the quinoa and oat flour, baking soda, and cinnamon in a medium bowl.
- Blend the egg, applesauce, and water in separate bowl.
- Fold the dry ingredients into the wet mixture and mix well. Fold the blueberries into the mixture.
- Pour the batter into a non-stick mini muffin pan, filling ½ full. Bake for 10 to 15 minutes.

Calories per Muffin: 20

So-Good Smoothies

Makes 8 smoothies

Blueberry Smoothie

½ cup blueberries   ½ cup plain non-fat yogurt

• Place the blueberries and yogurt in a blender. Blend on high until smooth. Evenly pour the mixture into 8 small paper cups.

Calories per Smoothie: 13

Strawberry Smoothie

½ cup strawberries   ½ cup plain non-fat yogurt

• Place the strawberries and yogurt in a blender. Blend on high until smooth. Evenly pour the mixture into 8 small paper cups.

Calories per Smoothie: 11

Pumpkin Smoothie

½ cup canned pumpkin   ½ cup plain non-fat yogurt

• Place the pumpkin and yogurt in a blender. Blend on high until smooth. Evenly pour the mixture into 8 small paper cups.

Calories per Smoothie: 13

Kitchen Hints & Tips

✓ These treats are great for soothing your pet's throat and gums after a dental cleaning.

✓ Most dogs love pumpkin. Try it and see.

Zucchini Tarts

Makes 24 tarts

¼ cup coconut flour

¼ teaspoon baking soda

1 teaspoon cinnamon

2 eggs

¼ cup applesauce

1½ cups grated zucchini

- Preheat the oven to 350°F.
- In a medium bowl, combine coconut flour, baking soda, and cinnamon.
- Add eggs, applesauce, and zucchini. Mix thoroughly.
- Generously spray a mini muffin pan with non-stick cooking spray and lighting dust with coconut flour. Evenly distribute the batter. Bake for 16 to 18 minutes. Cool.

Calories per Tart: 17 calories

 Kitchen Hints & Tips

✓ Coconut flour has a low glycemic index, is low in carbs, and is high in fiber. Coconut flour also contains 58% fiber compared to wheat bran, which contains only 27% fiber.

9

Rx 6:
Get Fido Fit

Most people treat exercise as something to be feared despite the fact that we were designed to move long distances often. Dogs and humans are arguably two of the most efficient and well-designed aerobic creatures on the planet. Much of our success as a species, even the development of human problem solving and intelligence, is directly related to our endurance.

Dogs are scavengers. They roam large distances searching for dead or dying prey. When they hunt, they typically form packs and bring down young or weak prey. One evolutionary theory is that dogs partnered with humans tens of thousands of years ago for survival. Each species had complementary skills; we ate the same foods and worked well in groups. If dogs had been unable to keep up with the early humans' nomadic ways, we never would have stayed together.

Engaging in physical activity together is an important component of the human-canine bond. Humans and dogs are the only two species that interrelate in this way. Try going for a four-mile jog with your cat sometime, and you'll fully appreciate what I mean. When we take out the aspect of physical interaction, the relationship is less than optimal. Dogs and people were designed to walk, run, and play side by side.

We've come a long way from our caveman days, and today's toy breeds would probably starve if forced to hunt, with or without human aid. What we haven't evolved from is this deeply rooted need to physically engage our dogs. Whether it's a walk or jog, throwing a ball or Frisbee, or a quiet evening stroll, these aspects of living with a dog are important.

Unfortunately, most modern dogs are inactive most of the day. In a 1977 study, beagles were observed to sleep or lay down in their cages 60 percent of each day. Tethered sled dogs were found to remain laying down 80 percent of the time in a 1986 study. Regardless of whether they were highly active or not, most dogs studied became largely inactive between 5 PM and 8 AM. Pet dogs also slept about half their day, according to a 1983 *Applied Animal Ethology* journal article. From my own experience, 50 percent seems a bit low even for my own dogs; they seem to sleep more like the sled dogs, only without the sled. A notable exception appears to be terrier breeds, which are known to stand much of the day. Perhaps for this reason we don't see as many obese Jack Russell and fox terriers.

The reality is that either by design or because of our lifestyle, pet dogs aren't exercising enough. While exercise isn't the only key to weight loss, it is a vital component of overall health and maintaining lean muscle mass.

Why Exercise Is Essential

Too many dog owners fail to understand that running and playing isn't just a by-product of health; it is a requirement for health. Dogs don't walk and run because they want to; they do it because they have to. The same is true for humans. We view exercise as something we do if we're able, instead of something we must do to remain healthy. Science has no better preventive measure for disease than aerobic exercise. Exercising your dog can prevent and treat cancer, heart disease, diabetes, arthritis, depression, anxiety, learning disorders, and more. What we need to ask is why? Why is aerobic activity so good for almost any ailment in dogs and people? The reason is that it is a vital component of our physiology. Dogs and humans run because we were made to run, just as we were made to breathe air and drink water. If humans don't breathe or drink or move enough, bad things begin to happen to our bodies and brains.

Dogs need it, too. Aerobic exercise keeps them healthy and makes them feel good. The first step in dealing with any behavioral problem is to increase activity and aerobic exercise. Everything from aggression to destruction to anxiety is treated, at least in part, with exercise. When dogs don't get regular exercise, they literally go crazy. Exercise is also essential for treating arthritis, heart disease, cancer, and so on. Exercise is the miracle cure so many people seek, yet disregard. If you want your dog to live a long and healthy life, exercise is essential.

Get Your Veterinarian's Blessing

If you think your dog is overweight, is over seven years of age, or has any preexisting problems such as arthritis, heart disease, or previous joint or back injuries, have your dog examined by your veterinarian before beginning an exercise program. It's also wise to get yourself checked, especially if it's been a while since you've been active. While most dogs with minor ailments have no problem participating in aerobic exercise, make sure your dog is healthy enough. In addition to a good physical examination, I recommend the following tests be performed before starting a weight-loss program.

- Complete physical examination and body condition scoring (BCS)
- Routine blood tests
  - CBC
  - Serum chemistries
  - Total thyroid hormone (T_4)

- Free T$_4$ by equilibrium dialysis
- Complete urinalysis
- Blood pressure
- Resting respiratory rate
- Resting heart rate
- Thoracic circumference (chest)
- Abdominal circumference (waist)
- Other tests as determined by your pet's condition
  - ECG
  - X-rays

When calculating how much your dog should exercise each day, consider how much and what types of physical activities your dog already does; its size, breed, and temperament; and its current diet. If you're reading this book, there's a good chance your dog needs additional exercise and (a lot) less food.

Power Walking for Pooches

Since one of the easiest activities to do is to walk with your dog, the first thing you should do is to mark off a one-mile course. This can be a stretch of road, a trail, or a track. If you typically walk a route in your neighborhood, drive your car and mark one mile from your normal starting point. On your next long walk, time how long it takes you and your dog to walk one mile. Don't push the pace; just walk at your normal speed. There will be plenty of time to speed things up in the future. Ultimately, your goal is to walk a "moderate," "target," or "excellent" pace for 30 minutes with your dog at least seven times a week. Depending upon your level of fitness and your dog's, this could take anywhere from a week to six weeks.

One-Mile Walk Time	Speed Zone
Greater than 22 minutes	S2 (Slow 2)
17 to 22 minutes	S1 (Slow 1)
16 to 17 minutes	M1 (Moderate 1)
15 to 16 minutes	M2 (Moderate 2)
14 to 15 minutes	T2 (Target 2)
13 to 14 minutes	T1 (Target 1)
12 to 13 minutes	E2 (Excellent)
Less than 12 minutes	E1 (Elite)

If you're slow, don't worry; you're not alone. In a study conducted in 2006 by the Association for Pet Obesity Prevention, we found that people walked their dogs at an average time of twenty-two minutes per mile. Why do people walk their dog so slowly? The answer is simple: that's the pace of a casual walker. The average human walks at a pace of about 3 miles per hour (twenty minutes per mile) and about 120 steps per minute. Most dogs, the exceptions being miniature and toy breeds, are comfortable walking at around 4 miles per hour or fifteen minutes per mile.

Unfortunately, if you walk at a slow pace (S1 to S2), it isn't going to help your dog lose weight or reap the physiological benefits of walking. At this pace, these dogs and their owners are *walking for pleasure,* which differs from *walking for exercise.* For example, my wife and I love to stroll along the beach in the evenings. We're not worried about our heart rate and we are engaged in conversation. This is walking for pleasure. Conversely, I run almost every morning for exercise. During my runs I am locked in to a specific heart rate zone, sweat profusely, and maintain a pace that makes talking difficult. This is *exercise.* Same movements, different objectives and benefits.

Walking with my wife has some health benefits. Most of them have to do with psychological as opposed to cardiovascular health. My morning runs, however, provide both psychological and physiological benefits. When it comes to walking your dog, you must adopt the same attitude. Some walks are for pleasure, and some walks are for exercise.

How Fast Should I Walk My Dog?

Clients always tell me, "I'm afraid I'll walk too fast for Fluffums." No way. It is very difficult to get a dog to exceed its aerobic limits during normal activities such as walking or running. This is one of the reasons that you seldom see elite runners running alongside their dog at a sub-six-minute-per-mile pace. Dogs can run that fast; they just don't see the need. If they were out hunting deer, well, that's a different story.

Think of aerobic activity as being long in duration yet low in intensity. This is just the type of activity your dog revels in. Aerobic exercise, such as briskly walking at a twelve- to fifteen-minute-per-mile pace, benefits you and your dog tremendously. And it helps you both lose weight.

Dogs love aerobic activity because they're extremely good at it. They're good at it because it's built into their muscle fibers. In numerous studies of dog muscle tissues, all of their muscle fibers were found to have a high aerobic capacity, were resistant to fatigue, and contained high concentrations of aerobic enzymes. The exercise physiology of dogs is very similar to that of humans, making us ideal companions.

We are also a good match in terms of speed and endurance. In a 1992 study published in the medical journal *Compendium*, scientists observed that trained sled dogs can maintain a speed of about 10 miles an hour, or a 6-minute-per-mile pace for ten to fourteen hours a day. That's flying! In comparison, the current record for the toughest (human) trail race, the Western States 100, is about 6.4 miles per hour over 100 miles of mountain passes, and world-record marathoners race at a 4:45-minute-per-mile pace.

How fast can your pooch go? The landmark study on dogs and maximum exercise was published in the *Journal of Applied Physiology*. Researchers from the University of Iowa and the U.S. Air Force Aerospace Medical Division set out to study the effects of exercise on untrained, trained, and cage-confined dogs.

To begin, the scientists found that almost any adult dog, regardless of previous exercise experience or level of fitness, had little trouble walking on a treadmill at 4 miles per hour. That's equal to a fifteen-minute-per-mile pace, or speed zone T2. At that pace the dogs experienced little change in heart rate or perceived exertion. To ensure the dog's safety on the treadmill, instead of speeding up, the researchers increased the incline of the treadmill. Once the dogs were walking at 4 miles an hour and at a 4 percent incline, their heart rates and exertion levels began to increase. Not excessively, but they finally entered into an aerobic training zone. On a flat road this effort would be approximately equal to just under a thirteen-minute-per-mile pace or about 4.7 miles per hour (E2). The dogs in the study gradually increased their incline to a staggering 20 percent, almost twice the steepest mountain grade in the Tour de France. All dogs in the study ran at the equivalent of just under an eight-minute-per-mile pace for three minutes as part of their training.

The dogs gradually increased their time until they were running for seventy-five minutes per day, five days per week. Three days a week they focused on slow, steep incline work to build endurance, and two days a week they worked on one-minute sprints and low inclines. The scientists found most dogs began to see improvement in their cardiovascular function in eight to ten weeks. What this means for your dog is that in two to three months, your lap potato can be well into the target zone (M1 to T2).

A Dog's Life

Just because dogs excel at aerobic activity doesn't mean your dog will go out and naturally select an aerobic pace. In fact, most dogs remain minimally active if allowed, like most adults I know. Our dogs are no dummies. If you're happy strolling along at two miles an hour, they'll happily follow. For our dogs to engage in healthy, persistent aerobic activity, it has to be fun and interactive. Too many dog owners mistakenly expect their dog to lead them. If you lead, they will follow. But often not without a nudge or three.

In numerous studies, dogs have been shown to remain largely inactive unless humans interact with them. In a 1992 *Applied Animal Behavioral* Science study, researchers found solitary dogs in a kennel setting were inactive 80 percent of the time. Can you blame them, being home alone with nothing to do but lay around? Dogs housed in groups still lay around a snooze-inducing 60 percent of the time.

Another good way to gauge your dog's pace is to count your footsteps per minute. Most people causally stroll at 96 to 110 steps per minute and walk at about 120 steps per minute. To begin to enter an aerobic-intensity zone, you'll need to approach 130 to 140 steps per minute, which is a brisk walk or slow jog for most people. Racewalking cadence begins at around 150 steps per minute. Most marathoners run at about 180 steps per minute—the most efficient cadence for running for most people. To quickly walk at a 140 steps per minute pace, you'll need to count about seventeen to eighteen left or right foot steps in a fifteen-second period.

Strive for an aerobic heart rate or around 130 to 140 steps per minute. Anything less is nice, just not as beneficial to your health as it could be. The bottom line is that if you are in an aerobic heart-rate zone, your dog probably is, too. You need to approach 4 miles per hour (fifteen minutes per mile) for your dog to experience the optimal health benefits of walking and for weight loss. Think of aerobic activity as being long in duration yet low in intensity. This is just the type of activity your dog revels in. Aerobic exercise, such as briskly walking at a twelve- to fifteen-minute-per-mile pace, benefits you and your dog tremendously. And it helps you both lose weight.

How Much Should I Exercise My Dog?

Unfortunately, you and your dog don't burn as many calories walking as you probably think. In general, dogs burn about 1.1 kcal/kg per kilometer trotting or running. This equals about 0.8 calories per pound per mile when the dog walks at a pace of 3.7 to 4 miles per hour. Interestingly, humans burn about 0.73 calories per pound per mile (1 kcal per kg per kilometer) on a treadmill. This means a 150 pound person will burn about 100 calories during 20 minutes of walking. If you examine this data closer, you'll find that, once again, dogs and humans are a perfect match. We both use about the same amount of energy walking and running on a level surface, making us excellent hunting, foraging, and exercise partners.

Weight of dog (lbs)	Distance walked (miles)	Approximate calories burned (kcals) at 3.7–4 mph pace (15–16 minutes per mile)
5	1	4
	2	8
	3	12
10	1	8
	2	16
	3	24
20	1	16
	2	32

Weight of dog (lbs)	Distance walked (miles)	Approximate calories burned (kcals) at 3.7–4 mph pace (15–16 minutes per mile)
(20 lb. dog continued)	3	48
40	1	32
	2	64
	3	96
60	1	48
	2	96
	3	144
80	1	64
	2	128
	3	192

In comparison to the chart, a 140-pound, 5'4" female would burn about 70 calories during twenty minutes of walking (one mile at 3 mph) or 79 calories in fifteen minutes (one mile at 4 mph).

If you walk your dog for thirty minutes a day at an average of 3.5 miles per hour, you cover about 1.75 miles. As the table illustrates, that's not going to burn a significant amount of calories. Remember that you and your dog must burn 3500 calories to shed one pound. Don't be discouraged, though, since you're walking your dog for other fitness and health benefits. And remember, in my experience, weight loss comes about 60 percent from diet and 40 percent from exercise.

If you want to increase the number of calories burned, you need to add distance, increase speed over the same period of time, or add resistance. Adding resistance is easiest achieved by walking uphill. Some people advocate the use of weighted vests in dogs to increase workload. I do not generally recommend this approach due to the concerns of overheating. Swimming is another way to burn calories, and both swimming and underwater treadmills are excellent options for dogs with arthritis and other joint problems.

Burn, Baby, Burn—Calories Burned by Walking

Weight of dog	Typical breeds	Suggested pace (minutes per mile)	Minimum distance walked per day
Less than 7 pounds	Chihuahua Japanese Chin Maltese Pomeranian Toy fox terrier Yorkshire terrier	20 to 25 (2.4 to 3.0 mph)	1 mile
7 to 10 pounds	American hairless terrier Affenpinscher Brussels Griffon Miniature pinscher Papillon Toy poodle	19 to 24 (2.5 to 3.2 mph)	1 mile
10 to 15 pounds	Bichon frise Cairn terrier Chinese crested Dachshund English toy spaniel Havanese Italian greyhound Jack Russell terrier Lhasa Apso Miniature poodle Pekingese Schipperke Shih Tzu Silky terrier Tibetan spaniel	17 to 23 (2.6 to 3.5 mph)	1½ miles
15 to 20 pounds	Boston terrier Cavalier King Charles spaniel Fox terrier Pug Welsh terrier West Highland white terrier	16 to 21 (2.7 to 3.7 mph)	2 miles

Burn, Baby Burn *(continued)*			
Weight of dog	Typical breeds	Suggested pace (minutes per mile)	Minimum distance walked per day
20 to 30 pounds	Basenji Beagle Cocker spaniel Pembroke Welsh corgi Scottish terrier Shetland sheepdog	15 to 20 (3.0 to 4.0 mph)	2½ miles
30 to 40 pounds	Australian Cattle Dog Border Collie Brittany Spaniel	12 to 18 (3.3 to 5.0 mph)	3 miles
Greater than 40 pounds	Basset hound Bulldog English springer spaniel Irish setter Golden retriever Labrador retriever Rottweiler	10 to 17 (3.5 to 6.0 mph)	More than 3 miles

Walking the Dog

It's your responsibility as a steward of good health to make your dog get its daily walk. Here are some tips to help you get started:

Get the Right Equipment

Harness Choice

Forget the leash and collar if you want to burn some serious calories with your dog. Collars can compress the trachea (windpipe) when pulled, causing difficulty breathing or even injury, and should be avoided. Especially risky are choke or pinch collars or constricting collars of any design. A walking harness (Ultra Paws Walking Harness, Gentle Leader Easy Walk, Sporn Simple Control Harness, and others) is your safest choice. Head halters provide you with the best control in the safest manner for dogs new to leash walking. An alternative is a no-pull harness, which offers you a higher degree of control than a traditional harness and is an alternative to a head halter for dogs that pull on a leash.

Look for wide, soft, and padded straps and breathable materials. The harness should fit snugly but not be too tight. You should be able to easily fit two fingers underneath the harness at all points. A well-designed harness distributes the force along the sternum or breast-bone area. This lower portion of the harness should be fairly wide to better disperse force. If you'll be walking your dog when it's warm outside, a mesh harness is ideal. The harness should be easy to adjust and the connector solid. A flimsy or cheap harness is not only uncomfortable for your dog but may lead to escape or injury.

Leash

When walking for exercise, I prefer leashes no longer than six feet, such as the EzyDog Leash. You'll be keeping your canine companion close to maintain a steady pace. Save the long leash and retractable gizmos for those casual strolls around the neighborhood when Fido wants to catch up on the latest pee-mail.

What If My Dog Pulls? What If I Can't Walk Him?

Many dog owners are embarrassed or scared to walk their dog around their neighborhood. They're afraid they'll be pulled off balance and fall down, or that their dog might bark, growl, or snap at a strange person or dog. These dogs rarely get any exercise and suffer the consequences of poor health. Worse, these dogs often develop behavioral issues because they're not getting adequate exercise. Every dog should be able to be leash-walked under control. If you can't walk your dog, there's only so much you can do to maintain their health. While there's no one-size-fits-all approach to teaching a dog to walk under control on a leash, here are some tips that may make your exercise more enjoyable.

1 Make sure you are in a calm and controlled state of mind before attempting to train your dog to leash-walk. If you're nervous or upset, your dog senses it and becomes anxious. An anxious dog is not able to focus and maintain attention. Further, if you're uncontrolled, you are more likely to snap or punish your dog if it doesn't respond properly. You dog will then become fearful and resist training the next time you attempt it. Dogs do not follow a person who they feel is not in control emotionally.

2 Click to win. Start with a short leash, head halter, and a clicker device. Have some tasty, low-cal food rewards available, such as tiny liver or salmon treats. The principle behind a clicker is that you "click" each time your dog does what you wish.

Clicker training goes something like this: Give your dog a command. When she follows it, click the device and offer praise and a treat. In this manner your dog associates the clicking sound with positive reinforcement and reward. Gradually reduce the food reward and rely on the clicker and praise.

The goal with this first exercise is to make training highly enjoyable for your dog. Think "calm, cool, and compassionate." Take your dog to a quiet part of your yard or house with minimal distractions.

Start by having your dog sit on your left side. Put the halter and leash on as you are giving your dog a treat. Constantly praise your dog and tell him how good he's being. Hold the leash in your right hand. Extend a treat with your left hand out in front of you to gently coax your dog to take a few steps. If you want to use a command such as "heel," say it calmly and at a normal volume as you offer the treat. Do not continue repeating the command. Saying it louder or more frequently does not cause your dog to respond any faster.

The leash should be kept slack as you guide your dog forward when you begin to walk. Take one to two steps and see if your dog follows. If it doesn't, try to lure him with the food. Don't jerk on the leash or pester the dog with "Heel, heel, HEEL!" Try to keep your dog's head just behind and to the side of your knee. After one or two steps with your dog close by your side, stop, click, praise, and give a tiny treat. Repeat often. Before long you'll be leash walking under control.

3 What if my dog pulls on the leash? If your dog lunges or doesn't stop when you do, don't jerk on the leash. If you pull on the leash, most dogs respond by pulling harder against you. This isn't a game of tug-of-war. It's better to discontinue the training if your dog won't comply. It's better to walk a few steps in the correct position than fail at a long walk before your dog is ready. Most dogs require two to five short sessions before you should attempt to walk them around the block.

As your dog gets better walking at your side, take a few more steps. You may find that holding a treat about thigh level may help your dog maintain the correct position. If it pulls the leash tight, stop and wait until the dog stops. Avoid giving commands such as, "No!" "Stop!" or "Bad!" These only serve to confuse your dog and may make them fearful of training. To correct a behavior, let your body do the talking. Because dogs communicate primarily through body language, they are keen on your every movement and gesture, however subtle it may seem to you.

A head halter helps you maintain control of a dog that surges or tugs. If your dog pulls ahead of you, the head halter will redirect its head so that it is turned toward you.

Your thoughts and emotions also influence how well your dog will walk with you. If you are confident and strong and signal, "You're not doing what I need you to do," your dog will understand this and respond. If your dog is being stubborn, practice visualizing exactly what you want your dog to do. Imagine your dog walking calmly by your side. You'll be surprised how your thoughts are translated into body movements your dog is able to read.

Remember you should not continue with the exercise or offer any reward until your dog complies. Your dog must learn what it should do rather than be forced to do it.

Once your dog stops or sits, click, praise, and reward. You always reward the stop or sit, even though that is not exactly the object of this exercise. Until your dog learns it will not be rewarded for pulling, you won't be able to proceed to controlled leash-walking.

4 Taking it to the streets. Once your dog is walking on a loose leash in your backyard or inside your house, it's time to take a test walk outside. Pick a time or day to begin when there are fewer distractions (people, cars, dogs, etc.). This exercise starts before you exit your house. Put your dog in a "sit and stay" position with your body between your dog and the door. Put on the head halter and leash and open the door. If your dog runs for the door, tighten the leash and give the "sit" command. As soon as your dog sits, click and reward. If she doesn't sit or continues to struggle for the door, you've got more work to do.

As your dog is sitting, let out a little slack in the leash and walk toward the door. If your dog gets up and bolts for the door again, repeat the "sit" command. If she calmly follows you, step through the door first (this is important; you must *always* lead your dog outside). This action gives your dog permission to follow you, not dash outdoors when she wants. As you are walking, don't let your dog walk in front of you; keep her head alongside your knee. As soon as you let your dog lead you, you've lost control. If it surges ahead, halt and don't move until it sits or stops. Reward it when it stops and continue. This may be repeated several times until your dog learns to walk just behind your left knee.

5 What if my dog refuses to walk? If your dog "puts on the brakes," most people make the mistake of dragging the dog along.

Even though it seems like the right thing to do, dragging never works. A dog's body is designed to resist being pulled forward. Think of a wolf gripping prey with its teeth. The front and rear legs extend forward, digging into the ground. The back and neck muscles tense. You think you're going to win this tug-of-war? Instead, use your intellect—and maybe a low-calorie goody—to try and coax it forward. Another option is to gently nudge your dog from the rear: push it forward. Once she resumes walking, reward and praise. It is imperative your dog enjoy walking on a leash, or you will always encounter challenges.

6 Take it easy. Gradually increase the amount of distractions your dog encounters when walking. Don't rush; it may take a few weeks to correctly train your dog to walk on a leash. The goal is to have a dog that allows you to lead it. Walking should be fun, exciting, and meaningful. Be sure to praise your dog liberally throughout training. With a little practice, you'll be surprised how well your once-unruly dog responds to strategic training techniques.

7 Walking on a loose leash. Walking for exercise requires both you and your dog to move at a brisk pace. You can't drag your dog along or stop and sit every five minutes. The ultimate goal is to be able to walk your dog on a loose or slack leash. Building on the techniques you've already learned, here are a few tips to help your dog become a speed walker right by your side.

While you are out walking, come to a complete stop. When your dog stops, click, praise, and reward. Let out three to four feet of leash; if your dog doesn't get up or walk away, give the command "Steady" in a low, calm voice. If it remains still, click, praise, and reward. If it gets up or walks away, give the "Steady" command and click, praise, and reward when it stops again.

Once your dog is relaxed, begin walking with the leash loose at your side. Your dog should resume its place behind your knee. If it pulls ahead, stop and repeat the training steps. Through repetition your dog learns that it is following you, not the leash. You are the control device, not the equipment.

Set the Right Pace

Based on observations of people walking with their dogs, the average pace is twenty-two minutes per mile. That is a slow troll with frequent pauses (on average every minute!) to allow their dog to smell an interesting object or mark territory. We're here to shed pounds, people, not smell the bushes!

Make your objective to walk briskly and focused on the outgoing leg of your walk, and then you can check the "pee-mail" on the return. I recommend starting the activity with the brisk or "hard" effort. Too often if we try to start slowly with the dog, allowing them to sniff and smell everything, we may have a challenging time getting them up to speed when we're ready. People often ask me, "Shouldn't we do a warm-up before we walk them?" I simply reply, "Have you ever seen a fox take a few warm-up laps before an all-out sprint to capture its prey?" Dogs are built to go from zero to maximum with very little risk of injury. And besides, you'll be going nowhere near an all-out sprint. If our dog's forefathers could see them now, what would they think? Of course, if you have an older pet or if your dog has an injury or medical condition, a short five-minute warm-up is a good idea.

Draw your leash close—generally within two to three feet of your body—and allow your dog to walk on a loose leash just behind your left knee or on the away-from-the-street side and set off at a pace you feel comfortable sustaining. This should be about a fifteen- to eighteen-minute-per-mile pace for most small to medium dogs. It should feel like a brisk walk, and you should break into a light sweat. The key is to keep it up. Your dog should understand that you have places to go, and this is different than your usual carefree, stop-and-smell-the-fire-hydrants affair.

The right pace should look like your dog is trotting alongside you. He should have a short stride and rapid leg turnover rate. Many dogs' legs appear almost as a blur when they are at their maximum efficiency. This fast leg turnover rate is essential to use less energy and maintain proper speed. As you focus on your own leg turnover rate, see how your dog adjusts to maintain speed. It is remarkable to watch such an efficient biomechanical system in motion.

What If My Dog Pants?

Another common reason clients cite for not walking briskly with their dog is panting. Dogs primarily breathe through an open mouth. In addition to breathing in oxygen and exhaling carbon dioxide, dogs breathe through their mouth to dissipate heat. Unlike humans, dogs have very few sweat glands to cool their body. If a dog didn't pant, it would quickly overheat. If you see your dog panting during a walk or trot, this is normal canine physiology in action. If your dog's breathing appears labored or noisy or if coughing develops, stop and check out your companion. Otherwise, admire the efficiency and grace with which your dog moves. Don't be overly alarmed if your dog is panting; this is no different than you breaking a sweat. If you're not sweating or your dog isn't panting, you're not working hard enough.

Set Time Goals

For most overweight or obese dogs that have normal heart and lung function, normal blood pressure, and no other preexisting medical conditions, I recommend starting with thirty-minute walks a minimum of five times per week. At first, don't worry as much about your speed or distance as your time. As you gain fitness, distance and pace become more important. A sample schedule follows:

	Long walk duration	Description
Week 1	30 minutes total	10 minutes brisk followed by 20 minutes casual pace
Week 2	30 minutes total	15 minutes brisk followed by 15 minutes casual pace
Week 3	30 minutes total	20 minutes brisk followed by 10 minutes casual pace
Week 4	35–40 minutes total	30 minutes brisk followed by 5–10 minutes casual pace
Week 5	35–45 minutes total each day	20- to 30-minute walks each day: 15–25 minutes brisk followed by 5–10 minutes casual pace
Week 6	30–60 minutes each day	Begin focusing on distance and pace: set a goal to walk one mile in 14 minutes or two miles in 30 minutes; cool down for 5–15 minutes on return. Begin adding one extra-long walk each week. Increase your time by 10 percent each week until you reach your desired long walk duration (i.e., one 60-minute walk each Sunday afternoon). Don't worry about pace or distance during your long walk; keep it as aerobic as possible. Long walks should be fun!

I encourage all dog owners to walk with their dog thirty minutes every day if possible after they become comfortable with "real walking." The health benefits for you and your pet are simply incredible!

The Extra-Long Walk

Occasionally you may find that due to unexpected occurrences, you may miss one or two walks during the week. Don't fret. You can gain back some of the benefits by adding on a longer, slower walk during the weekend. Whenever possible, even if you're able to walk every day for thirty or more minutes, try to go for a longer period at least once a week. For many dog owners this means an hour-long hike or more casual walk on the weekends. For these activities, a less intense pace of 120 steps per minute or seventeen to twenty minutes per mile is fine. Of course, as your fitness improves, you'll find yourself walking faster. In addition to improving aerobic fitness, these longer walks also help burn additional calories. However, don't make the big mistake and reward your dog with food treats after a long walk.

I've had too many weight-loss clients complain that their dog doesn't lose weight despite strict adherence to my exercise plan. The usual culprit: feeding their dog more, especially after a long walk. Overfeeding is generally due to the "justification factor." People think their dog "earned" an extra treat because it exercised for a long time. That might be true, if your dog didn't need to lose weight. Don't make this rookie mistake and then wonder why your dog is still overweight.

Check the Paws

Once you've begun a regular walking program with your dog, inspect its footpads for any injuries or problems. Check also that the nails are short and healthy.

Weather and Environmental Issues

Chill Out When It Gets Too Hot

The amount of time a dog can exercise in the heat depends on several factors: the acclimatization of the dog (how long and frequently it has been exposed to hot temperatures), its current fitness levels (lean, fitter dogs can endure high temperatures longer than out-of-shape, overweight dogs), and hydration status.

In general, once it gets above 85 degrees Fahrenheit, dog owners should use caution when exercising their dog outdoors. For most dogs, moderate activity for thirty minutes is safe. When temperatures exceed

95 degrees, skip the outdoor workout until it cools down. During the summer months, try to walk or jog in the early morning or evenings or seek shady trails.

If your dog begins to have rapid or labored breathing, begins to resist walking, or acts depressed, your dog may be overheating. In these cases, stop, rest, and rehydrate. Don't cease exercising just because your dog is panting; you need to closely watch your pet to determine if the panting is excessive or abnormal. If in doubt, take a break and cool down. According to a *Journal of Nutrition* study, most dogs can fully recover within nine minutes after exertion.

Stay Hydrated

Pets that play or spend time outdoors in the heat need to drink plenty of water. A dog that becomes 5 percent dehydrated develops early signs of heat stress, while a pet that experiences 10 percent dehydration is severely ill and requires immediate medical assistance. To avoid dehydration, always carry fresh water with you when it's hot or if you're out for a long walk. Be sure to offer water to your dog at least every thirty minutes. Many styles of portable dog bowls are convenient to carry. Under normal circumstances, most pets drink about an ounce of water per pound of body weight per day. In hot and humid conditions, your pet may need three to four times this amount.

Dogs Get Sunburned, Too

Dogs are susceptible to the same damage from ultraviolet rays as humans, especially white or light-colored pets. Particularly at risk are areas of the body that are thinly haired, such as the nose, face, and ears, and breeds with little hair such as Shar Peis and Chinese crested hairless dogs. Dog sun suits, visors, and hats can protect at-risk dogs and are available in a variety of designs, colors, and materials to suit an individual's preference. Look for a suit that is at least 30+ UPF, with 50+ UPF ideal.

The eyes and nose of dogs are highly susceptible to damage from the sun's rays because they are typically lightly pigmented and frequently exposed to direct sunlight. I recommend using a children's sunscreen that contains avobenzone, also called Parsol 1789, which is a UVA blocker, and octisalate, which blocks UVB rays. Avoid sunscreens that contain zinc oxide because accidental ingestion could lead to a serious condition called hemolytic anemia in some pets.

Treadmills

Doggy treadmills are great "no excuse" tools for exercising your dog. Treadmills are fantastic for rehab after injury, weight loss, dogs with arthritis, and those that live in high-rise apartments or with owners who have physical limitations or whose schedules don't permit daily exercise.

Walking on a treadmill is different than walking your dog outdoors. This isn't an activity that you can simply hook your pet onto the treadmill and walk away. A pet tethered to a treadmill could fall and seriously injure itself. You'll need to closely supervise your pet for any signs of fatigue, discomfort, or shortness of breath. *Never* attach your dog to a treadmill or leave it unattended.

Start with the treadmill off and at a 0 percent incline in a well-ventilated area. I recommend placing a nonslip rug behind the treadmill to cushion any inadvertent falls and to prevent slipping when exiting the treadmill. Use a walking harness with a front hook attached to a short leash to guide your dog onto the treadmill. Coax your dog onto the platform with generous praise. Be sure to start the treadmill at its slowest setting. As your dog gets used to walking on the moving surface, you can increase the speed and incline until your dog appears to be at a brisk, yet comfortable, sustainable pace. Begin the walks for five minutes with a two- to three-minute break and repeat. As your dog develops aerobic fitness, you may increase the time without stopping to twenty to thirty minutes. Once your dog is comfortable trotting on the treadmill at 4 miles per hour, increase the incline to challenge your dog and gain improved strength and endurance.

Environmental Enrichment

In its most basic form, behavioral enrichment means changing things in the surroundings to keep it fresh and interesting: adding a new obstacle, a play toy, or a feature such as a ramp or obstacles are all examples of environmental enrichment.

You can add excitement to your dog's daily dull dash by using the same principle. Try these ideas:

- Try hiding treats in corners of your yard, under bushes, or on the side of a tree within reach.
- Buy an obstacle course or agility equipment (and teach your dogs to use it, with you, of course).
- Make unexpected forays into your backyard to throw a favorite ball or toy before returning inside.
- Get a wading pool for use in the summer.
- Rotate your dog's toys, allowing access for only a day or two before putting one away and swapping out for another.
- Use toys that require concentration and problem-solving such as food puzzles or treats stuffed inside interactive toys. Use electronic or remote-controlled toys. There are now motion-activated dog toys that talk when they sense your dog's presence, even breathing. Some roll, vibrate, or move when your dog picks it up. Others blink a flashing light.

You can provide an endless variety of environmental enrichments for your dog. While none can replace the power of personal interaction, for time-pressed dog owners, these ideas can make a difference over time. Anything that gets your dog mentally and physically motivated will help it be healthier and happier.

You–the Best Dog Toy

Numerous studies show that dogs remain largely inactive unless humans interact with them. Several years ago I had a client who insisted she couldn't walk or play with her overweight dog; she was simply too busy. I asked her to help me with a little experiment. She was eager to try anything that removed her from the responsibility of exercising her dog. I had record her voice on a tape player saying every five minutes, "Cody, come here! Here, Cody, here!" She then put Cody outside and played the tape. I wish I could say the experiment was a success. At first, when Cody heard his name he bounded to source of the sound. Confused when he didn't see his owner, he quickly returned to sniffing in the yard. After three or four times repeating this process, Cody stopped coming. We never made it to Day Two. She never walked Cody or put him on a diet, and he became terribly obese in his later years. It just goes to show how important the physical and mental connection between us and our dogs really is. Cody wanted to come because he wanted to play with his owner. Once he realized it was a vacant promise, he quit. Can't say I blame him.

Aerobic Exercise and Games

When it comes to fun and weight loss for dogs, outdoor play can't be beat. To keep it entertaining and to ramp up the number of calories you're burning, try some of these activities with your dog the next time you go for some exercise:

Fetch!

One of the most entertaining activities for most dogs is fetch. Many dogs instinctively retrieve thrown objects with little training. Playing fetch requires you to train your dog to do three actions: go after the toy, return the toy, and give the toy back to you. The first two are easy for most dogs; giving the toy back is a deal-breaker for many dogs. "I did all that work and it's mine!" they seem to be saying as they run away, ball in mouth. Here are some suggestions for making the game of fetch productive and fun.

Use a fun toy. Many dogs won't retrieve just any old thing. Make sure the toy you use to train your dog is one that your dog likes. Just because the package says, "Fun!" doesn't mean your dog agrees.

Get your dog's attention. Show your dog the toy. Make funny noises to get its attention. Make sure your dog is following the toy in your hands. I believe in displaying "play" body language prior to starting a game such as fetch. Bend over and extend your arms down and out as if bowing to your dog. If you've ever watched two dogs play together, you'll see this posture before they launch at each other's throats. This important signal is the way dogs tell each other, "Okay, I'm ready to play. Everything that follows is for fun, not for fighting."

Start with baby throws. Once you have your dog's attention, throw the ball or toy a couple of feet away. When your dog reaches the thrown toy, click and praise. If your dog picks up the toy with its mouth, click and praise generously. As soon as it puts the toy in its mouth, take a few steps away while calling your dog to you. As your dog begins to walk toward you, continue offering praise. When your dog reaches you, give the command "Release" and show it a treat. The majority of dogs will trade the toy for a goody. As soon as your dog drops the toy, click, praise, and reward. Repeat this sequence many times, each time throwing the toy a little farther. Before you know it, your dog will be a champion retriever!

If your dog doesn't retrieve the toy. If your dog doesn't go for the toy immediately, encourage it to move to the toy. When your dog reaches the toy, put it in your dog's mouth. Click and praise your dog. While the toy is still in the dog's mouth, take a few steps away. Call your dog to you. Once it reaches you, show it a treat and say, "Release." As soon as your dog drops the toy, click, praise, and give it the treat.

If your dog doesn't give the toy back.

Some dogs like to play "chase" more than "fetch." For these dogs, try using two favorite toys in your game of fetch. Throw one toy and as your dog is returning it to you, show it the other toy. Tell your dog, "Release," as you wave the second toy in your hand. As soon as it drops the toy, click, praise, and throw the second toy. Pick up the first toy and repeat. After practicing this for several sessions, most dogs learn to play fetch with one toy.

Playing with two dogs.

If you're playing fetch with two dogs and one toy, competition can occur. Some dogs play well together while others need to always get the toy. If one dog is dominating a game of fetch, if the two dogs are of different sizes or abilities, or if they simply don't play well together, try using two toys. Throw each toy in opposite directions. You may find that staggering your throws or throwing them close together works best for you. Whatever you do, don't allow one dog to monopolize the game or intimidate the other. If this occurs, the losing dog may become frustrated and either stop playing or turn aggressive.

Always get the toy in the end.

It is important that you always take the toy at the end of each session of fetch. If you don't, your dog may decide it enjoys "see-if-you-can-take-it-from me" better.

Come and Get It!

This game takes place in a backyard or park. With your dog off-leash, get its attention by making a noise. Show your dog a favorite toy such as ball or Frisbee. As you do this, quickly bend over at the waist and extend your arms downward. This nonverbal communication cue signals you want to play. While you're bending over, say, "Come and get it!" As soon as you're certain you've gotten your dog's attention, turn and run away. As soon as your dog gets within three or four feet, stop and offer praise and a treat reward. Stop before your dog reaches you or he may try to nip at your leg. If your dog isn't interested in chasing you, don't chase the dog, which may inadvertently teach your dog that it's a game to run from you.

Make sure you give your dog the toy if you use it as a reward. Dogs can become frustrated if they try to get it and never succeed. After ten or fifteen minutes, it's usually time to move on to another game.

Fast and Slow

Interval training or mixing in short bursts of speed during a slower activity is a great way to spark a lagging metabolism. When preparing for a triathlon, it is common to do interval training in the pool, on the bike, and on the track at least once a week. By varying speed and intensity, triathletes recruit different muscle fibers and utilize different energy systems. For dogs, I recommend going fast for three minutes and then easy for three minutes during a normal twenty- or thirty-minute walk. For example, walk at a 140- to 150-steps-per-minute or fourteen- to fifteen-minute-per-mile pace for about two blocks or three minutes, then 110 to 120 steps per minute for three minutes. If that is uncomfortable for you, try walking at the faster pace for a minute or two until your fitness improves. Your dog will love the unexpected surges, and it will fire up a smoldering weight-loss program. Do this once or twice a week during your normal twenty- to thirty-minute walks.

Obstacle Course

In your backyard, try setting up a basic agility or obstacle course. My favorite fun fitness device is a climbing obstacle or ramp. You can purchase these online or at a pet store. Teach your dog to climb up the ramp by slowly guiding it with a leash and treat. Clicker training is also very helpful in training dogs to navigate an obstacle course. Climbing up and down uses your dog's largest muscle masses in the rear legs. When the hamstrings (back of the leg) and quadriceps (thigh muscles) are engaged, your dog is burning calories. Weaving poles and jumping bars are also great ways to make exercise fun for your dog. Dogs want to learn new skills, just like we do. Teaching old dogs new tricks can not only help then lose weight, but also help them stay mentally healthy as well.

Stair Mutts and Hill Hounds

Stairs can be a fantastic way to tone muscle and burn fat in dogs. Before you walk your dogs on stairs or hills, make sure your veterinarian has carefully evaluated your dog's knees and hips. Obese dogs can put more stress on their joints, resulting in higher frequency of injuries.

Just because your dog is too heavy doesn't mean it can't walk up and down stairs or trot uphill. Most dogs exercise at slow speeds. The majority of injuries occur when a dog sprints or makes a sudden turn or abrupt stop. As long as you keep these activities controlled, you should be fine. Many veterinarians and physicians fear steps and hills because they don't properly understand them. In human weight loss, maintaining a slow speed and increasing the incline when doing treadmill workouts is often preferable to flatter, faster speeds. Cardiac stress tests also employ this technique. Don't fear gradients; use them as part of a complete and balanced exercise program for you and your dog.

A simple technique for healthy overweight dogs is to find a hilly trail or flight of stairs and walk up and down. Maintain a moderate pace and avoid sharp turns or jumps. Five to ten minutes of solid hill or stair climbing is a great workout for any pudgy person or pooch.

If you have easy access to stairs or hills, try using them as often as possible. Inclines use more leg muscles than walking or running on flat ground.

Swimming

You won't have to enroll your dog in swim classes because all dogs can swim, some better than others. Many breeds, such as retrievers, seem hard-wired to dive in and go. If your dog likes to swim, indulge.

If you're planning on diving into a local swimming hole, watch out for snakes, alligators, fire ants, and wasps in the surrounding area. Know if the pond contains chemicals or sewage before you allow your dog to jump in. Be aware that hidden dangers may lurk below the surface, such as drainage pipes, debris, and plants. Ask people who live nearby if they know about the lake or pond. Check to make sure it's legal for your dog to swim in the lake. Don't let your dog drink the water unless you're certain it's safe. Dogs will also drink saltwater and then experience vomiting and diarrhea.

If your dog has a history of joint injuries or arthritis, swimming is an excellent exercise option. Swimming is a great no-impact activity in which a dog in almost any condition can participate.

Indoor Games

Not every day can be an outdoor play day. Rain, heat, snow, and wind can all sidetrack an exercise program. Even though the weather is bad, you still need to exercise your dog. While indoor activities, with the exception of treadmill walking, may not be as intense as outdoor exercise, they still serve a valuable purpose. Indoor play can keep your dog stimulated, preventing unwanted or destructive behavior. Even a few minutes of play can raise your dog's heart rate enough to burn off at least a few calories.

Over the years a common excuse has been, "We'll start walking as soon as it warms up." This excuse is followed by, "It's just been too hot to do much walking." Regardless of the weather, you still owe your dog play time. Use these indoor games as starters for play time with your dog the next time you're confined due to inclement weather.

Hide and Seek

This is similar to fetch but without the running and throwing (and broken lamps). Show your dog one of its favorite toys. Have someone take the dog into another room or hide the toy from your dog's view. Place the toy under a cushion or pillow. Make it easy and obvious at first. When your dog finds it, click, praise, and give a treat. Hide the toy in progressively more challenging places as the game continues.

High and Low

This game is similar to squats or plyometrics with your dog (and it can also be played outside). With a small piece of treat in one hand, have your dog lie down or sit. Lower the treat and coax your dog to jump up and follow the treat. Quickly lower the treat and return the dog to a sitting or lying position. Repeat this three to five times before giving your dog the tiny treat. An ideal "high and low" is when your dog explodes upward and immediately lays down again. Do this activity for five to ten minutes, and your dog will get a good workout.

Follow the Leader

This classic indoor game uses the same skills as "come and get it." Show your dog a favorite toy and call her to you. Walk around your house with your dog following you.

Remote-Controlled Toys

Technology has provided dog owners an almost endless supply of remote-controlled toys. Many dogs will chase a remote-controlled car or interactive talking toy. Look for a dog-friendly toy or car that has few small parts or is durable enough to withstand a paw strike or bite. Don't scold your dog if it destroys the toy; it happens.

•   •   •

Exercising your dog can be as basic as walking around the block or as complex as an agility-course competition. Find an activity that suits both you and your dog and do it consistently. Add new routes, games, and toys on a regular basis. Exercise, while it certainly won't replace feeding fewer calories when it comes to your dog losing weight, is a vital part of a healthy lifestyle for both humans and dogs. When you and your pet move together, you celebrate one of the oldest, most unique, and most extraordinary bonds our planet has ever known.

10

Rx 7:
Track Your Progress

"Whate gets measured gets done." This statement is particularly important when dealing with diet and exercise.
A 2006 Centers for Disease Control study proved that people who
record their activities and diet remain with weight-loss programs and
develop healthier lifestyles sooner than those who don't. Of over 6,000
weight-loss participants, those who tracked their activities and meals
had a higher rate of maintaining lower weight and experiencing less
weight regain, and they continued exercise programs longer. In
summary, the CDC scientists concluded that self-tracking was an
important aspect of maintaining a healthy weight and avoiding yo-
yo dieting.

The same is true when beginning a weight-loss program for your
dog. If you record the most basic data for a few weeks, before long you
will have changed your behavior. You will have gained a sense of what
and how much you should feed and when you've exercised enough.

Another key element of an activity and diet log is accountability.
When you know you'll have to write down those two extra treats,
you're less likely to give them to your dog. You'll feel guilty when you
have to enter "zero" for your daily walk when you (and your dog) know
you needed to walk thirty minutes. A written log, in paper or online,

is a great way not only to track your progress but also to confront your setbacks. The act of transferring to a journal what you did or didn't do is a powerful motivator.

Keep It Simple

The key elements to track are how much and what you fed your dog, how many and what type of treats you gave, and how long you walked or played each day. That's it. If you want to go into information overdrive, great, go ahead. Whatever you do, pick elements you can consistently and accurately measure.

Table 10.1. Sample Diet and Activity Log

Date and Time	Food/Cals	Treats/Cals	Activity	Notes	Total Calories for the Day	Total Exercise Time for the Day
Day 1 8 AM	½ cup Happy Dog Food 175 cal	2 Happy Dog Treats 50 cal	Bathroom duty— no walk	Raining outside		
12:30 PM		2 Happy Dog Treats 50 cal	5-minute walk			
6:00 PM	½ cup Happy Dog Food 175 cal	2 Happy Dog Treats 50 cal Small piece of leftover chicken breast 25 cal	20-minute walk		425	25 minutes

Evaluate Your Dog's Lifestyle

The first step in weight loss for your dog is to determine where you currently are in terms of diet and exercise. Before you change anything, record your daily feedings and activities. The simple act of recording may slightly alter what you do with your dog, but it will give you a good idea of what you're doing.

After a week, count the number of calories you're feeding and the number of minutes you're exercising with your dog each day. For many dog owners, especially those with heavy dogs, you'll find you're feeding too much and moving too little. No worries; these problems are easily corrected.

The most important and hardest part of evaluating your current lifestyle is being honest. Too often dog owners soften their answers to make the situation appear better than it really is. This is human nature. In another 2006 Centers for Disease Control study, 70 percent of obese people reported they ate "a healthy diet," and 40 percent stated they participated in twenty minutes of "vigorous exercise" at least three times a week. When people are asked questions about their lifestyle, they often embellish.

This isn't the time for exaggeration. If your dog is overweight, there's a reason. That reason usually involves eating too much and exercising too little. You must transcend yourself and focus on your dog's health. Many dog owners see their dog's weight as a reflection of their own laziness or poor care. Still others view any discussion of their pet's weight as an attack on their own weight or lifestyle. The issue has nothing to do with you, the dog owner. If you feel offended or angered by someone pointing out your dog's excess weight, the issue lies within yourself, not the other person. Keep the focus on your dog's health, and everyone benefits.

The First Month Is the Hardest

Our goal with health and fitness is to develop a healthy lifestyle we can continue for the rest of our dog's life. Eating a healthy, balanced diet and engaging in daily aerobic activity become second nature for us and our dog. This healthy lifestyle evolves into something natural to us, a habit. Ultimately, you can't imagine a time when you didn't eat for health and exercise daily.

Unfortunately, getting to "second nature" and "habit" can seem infinitely far away when you're starting out. A common question posed by dog owners and participants in lifestyle change is, "How long will it take?" That question is the wrong one to ask. The answer varies from individual to individual and the amount of change each is seeking to undertake. Someone attempting to quit smoking may take months to acquire the "habit" of not smoking, while a person who desires to walk thirty minutes five days a week may find it is a part of their routine within three weeks.

Instead of focusing on "How long will take to become easy?" focus instead on small, achievable goals. Make it your goal to walk your dog every day, rain or shine, for the next month. At the end of the month, celebrate by going to a special dog park or beach, or enjoy a long hike.

During the first month of your dog's weight-loss program, you should strive to eliminate all processed dog treats. This means no dog bones or chews—anything that's full of carbohydrates, fat, and sugar. The only treats you should give your dog are healthy vegetables, ice, and other low-calorie nutritious snacks.

Pre-Program	Record your current diet and activity for one week.
Step 1	Calculate the number of calories your dog needs per day.
Step 2	Eliminate snacks except vegetables, healthy treats, and ice.
Step 3	Begin a structured daily exercise program.
Step 4	Weigh monthly.
Step 5	Adjust calories and exercise as needed.
Step 6	Change tactics in three months if appreciable weight loss and improved fitness are not observed.

The first month should be about changing into a new lifestyle. You must discard the old, high-calorie lifestyle and embrace the new, nutritious way of life. Dr. Dean Ornish has published numerous medical studies demonstrating that major, abrupt changes are often best when it comes to diet and lifestyle in people confronting heart disease, smoking, and obesity. If you set out to help your dog lose weight, do it. The first month is the hardest because you'll be met with pleading eyes, plaintive wails, and looks of extreme disappointment from your best friend. Guilt quickly follows, and it's not long before you're reaching for salty, sugary, and fatty snacks for your dog. Keep in mind that your dog is, in many ways, addicted to food. The first month is about retraining both your and your dog's behavior and how you both use food as part of your daily routine—in good and bad ways.

Every time you're feeling the need to give an extra goody, pause. Remember that your dog wants you—your time, affection, and interaction—more than any doggy delicacy. Give them what they want most before giving them what is easiest and accessible. By replacing *confection* with *affection*, you'll be developing healthy habits that leave you both satisfied and healthy.

Weigh your dog monthly. Any sooner and you probably won't see enough results to be appreciated. Of course, if you can and are able to weigh your dog weekly, do so. I caution you against chasing week-to-week results for fear you may miss a larger trend. For example, some dog owners become discouraged if their dog fails to lose weight for two or three consecutive weeks. I am cautious at this stage, but not pessimistic. I typically recommend evaluating weight loss and fitness gains not in terms of weeks but months, generally a three-month period. If things aren't working within three months, it's time to change something in your program.

> **❝ Remember that your dog wants you—your time, affection, and interaction—more than any doggy delicacy. . . . By replacing confection with affection, you'll be developing healthy habits that leave you both satisfied and healthy. ❞**

Typically after two to three months of recording your daily activities, you begin to fall into new behavior patterns. You may start to relax some of your daily data entry as healthy habits become a natural part of your routine. If you miss a workout, you start to feel edgy. That doesn't mean you need to double the time of your next activity, just continue with your normal schedule. The key is to not let one missed day of exercise lead to two, and then suddenly a week has gone by without much activity. Skipping exercise is a seductive proposition; you can create almost endless excuses for not breaking a sweat. Once you begin rationalizing away your healthy diet and exercise, it's hard to regain momentum.

One of the keys to my years of successful triathlon racing has been the fact that I religiously track everything. Technology certainly makes this easier today than five or ten years ago. Today's gadgets sync with your computer to record all pertinent workout data. You can then view your week, month, or year and see if you're faster, more fit, or holding steady. What gets measured gets done. The same is true with your dog's health.

11

TROUBLESHOOTING:
Plateaus, Pestering, and Other Problems

Albert Einstein is attributed with saying, "Insanity is doing the same thing over and over again and expecting different results." It is highly unlikely that Einstein was thinking of pet obesity when he made this statement. His observation applies directly to what many adults and dog owners experience when they struggle with weight loss. The common refrain, "I've been [eating/feeding] this diet for six months and [I don't/my pet doesn't] seem to be losing weight," can be heard in gyms, doctor's offices, and veterinary clinics world-wide. The sad reality is that people say this and yet continue in their set ways. Whatever they're doing isn't working, yet they persist, expecting something to change. It's insanity.

What Happens When the Diet Isn't Working

Many overweight dogs experience some mild to moderate weight loss initially and then stop losing weight. They've encountered the dreaded plateau. Most people who've started a fad diet know this pattern too well: Start the diet, lose weight, and everything's great. Weight loss stops, diet is hard to maintain, regain weight. This is the definition of yo-yo dieting. You'd be surprised at the number of yo-yo dogs I see.

How do you get your dog off the weight-loss roller-coaster? Better yet, how do you avoid the roller-coaster altogether?

First, accept that you may encounter challenges when you begin a weight-loss program. Not every dog that starts a weight-loss program has the same results. Some lose weight easily and quickly, and others lose it slowly and with much strife. The question shouldn't be, "How long will it take?" but rather, "How much healthier will my dog be?" I recommend that you focus on improving health instead of chasing a number on a scale.

What happens when you've been doing exactly what your veterinarian asked you to do and your dog isn't losing weight? You may have to take greater charge in this case. If something isn't giving you the results you desire—in this case, weight loss—change it. If you don't change something, nothing will change.

The Ninety-Day Rule:
When Your Dog Isn't Making Progress

For dog owners needing a simple rule to diet by, here it is: if your dog isn't losing appreciable weight in ninety days of starting a diet or exercise program, change it.

The first change is the amount of calories you're feeding. If you're feeding your dog its daily resting energy requirement (RER), reduce it to 80 percent RER. I typically do not recommend lowering your dog's calories below 70 percent RER unless your veterinarian specifically authorizes it. Keep in mind that when you're lowering calories, you're also reducing essential nutrients. If you feed too little of a diet, your dog could, although rarely, develop nutritional deficiencies. Weight loss isn't about starvation or deprivation; it's about a strategic approach to altering your dog's calorie intake while maintaining optimal health.

If you're already feeding 70 percent RER, change diets. If you were feeding a high-protein, low-calorie diet, try a high-fiber approach. Mix it up. Every dog's (and person's) metabolism works differently. The goal is to find an approach that works best for your pet and lifestyle.

In addition to changing to the nutrient formulation, I often recommend changing brands when my patients aren't achieving target weights and following my "no treats" rule. You should try different brands, because many companies espouse a nutritional philosophy carried throughout their product line. Each dog food manufacturer has preferred protein, carbohydrate, and fat sources. If your dog does well on a brand's food, stick with it. If not, find an alternative. Do not allow your dog to be locked into a specific brand or line of food unless it is providing optimal health for your dog.

The 60:40 Rule

Diet is the primary driver of weight loss. Exercise is a key ingredient but not as important as calories. For many years, I've shared with my human and veterinary weight-loss patients a weight-loss rule I began observing years ago: Weight loss is about 60 percent diet and 40 percent exercise, which means you and your dog can lose a ton of weight without ever walking a step.

Many people instantly put up the "I don't have time to exercise" defense when I mention weight loss. You don't have to exercise your dog much to help him lose excess pounds or maintain a healthy weight. The benefits of exercise extend far beyond that of the scale; exercise promotes health and prevents disease by engaging physical and biochemical processes separate from your diet. I don't think anyone or any dog can achieve optimal health without routine aerobic activity. You and your dog are healthier because you exercise.

By enacting the 60:40 Rule, the balance is clearly tipped in favor of calories consumed versus calories burned.

I wasn't the only one who made this observation. In the February 18, 2009, issue of the *Public Library of Science ONE* journal, Dr.

Timothy Church and colleagues followed 464 overweight women for six months. The women were divided into four groups: one with no exercise or change in diet and the other three with increasing levels of exercise. Sadly, no one really lost weight during the study. I say sadly because the study was examining how much exercise to recommend for weight loss. Instead, this widely publicized study illustrated how little impact exercise has on weight loss. These overweight women were only exercising for a maximum of just over three hours a week, so it's no big surprise significant weight loss wasn't observed. However, when you compare the no-diet and no-exercise group with the no-diet and exercise group, you can't help but feeling a little cheated.

Break the Reward Rule

Many personal trainers and physicians know the key reason these women failed to lose weight: the Reward Rule. Many people who run an extra mile or swim an extra ten minutes feel entitled to a reward. We believe we've "earned" that extra muffin or caffe latte. We over-estimate the number of calories we've burned during our workout (that extra mile only netted you about 100 calories or a third of a muffin) and rationalize an indulgence as already paid for with hard work. As reported in the May 2008 issue of the *International Journal of Obesity*, researchers from Harvard University followed 538 school-aged boys for two years. They found that as their subjects exercised more, they began to eat more. In fact, they were surprised to find that the boys ate more than 100 calories more than they burned during exercise.

The take-home message from the Harvard study is that we must take heed not to eat more than we're burning, which extends also to our four-legged friends. Because most of my clients are exercising alongside their dogs and they are also trying to lose or maintain weight, the Reward Rule comes into play. A dog owner who feels entitled to a reward and shares it with his dog can torpedo a beneficial workout with as few as two doggie treats or one blueberry muffin. If you don't think so, check out the chart below, which shows the human equivalent of the calorie damage by even just a few small rewards.

10-pound Dog _Requiring 200 to 220 Calories Per Day_			
If Your Dog Eats This . . .	**Number of Calories**	**It's Like You Eating That . . .**	**Number of Calories**
¼ slice Pizza Hut Pepperoni Pizza	50	3 slices Pizza Hut Pepperoni Pizza	600
1 tablespoon Ben & Jerry's Vanilla Ice Cream	30	¾ cup Ben & Jerry's Vanilla Ice Cream	320
1 cube Kraft Natural Cube Cheese Choddar (Mild)	15	1 1-ounce bag Flamin' Hot Lays potato chips	160
1 animal cracker	11	1 box animal crackers	130
1 ginger snap	29	11 ginger snaps	319
½ sugar cookie from refrigerated dough	55	5½ sugar cookies from refrigerated dough	611
½ Oscar Meyer Beef Frank (Hot Dog Weiner)	74	3 plain hot dogs with ketchup and mustard	726
1 regular marshmallow	23	11 regular marshmallows	230
1 tortilla chip (Tostitos)	11	11 tortilla chips	121
1 oz. of an 8-oz. broiled T-bone steak—¼" trim (⅛ of steak, approx 1–1.5" cube)	87	2 regular cheeseburgers and 8 oz. chocolate shake	957 (718+239)
½ slice toast (white bread)	40	5½ slices toast (white bread)	440

Based on a 2300 calories-per-day human diet

20-pound Dog Requiring 340 to 360 Calories Per Day			
If Your Dog Eats This . . .	**Number of Calories**	**It's Like You Eating That . . .**	**Number of Calories**
2 Nabisco Premium Saltines crackers	24	1 Dunkin' Donuts French Cruller	150
1 Fig Newton	55	7 Fig Newtons	385
½ slice white bread	40	6-inch Subway Turkey Breast Sandwich	280
½ Oscar Meyer Beef Frank (Hot Dog Weiner)	74	1 8-oz. Choice, Lean Broiled T-bone Steak	465
¼ slice Domino's Hand Tossed Cheese Pizza— Large pizza	73	1¾ slices Domino's Hand Tossed Cheese Pizza— Large pizza	511
¼ plain bagel (3½" diameter)	72	4 homemade brownies (2" square)	448
1 slice pan-fried bacon	43	6½ slices pan-fried bacon	280
1 slice toast (white bread)	80	6½ slices toast (white bread)	520

Based on a 2300 calories-per-day human diet

40-pound Dog
Requiring 620 to 650 Calories Per Day

If Your Dog Eats This ...	Number of Calories	It's Like You Eating That ...	Number of Calories
1 regular marshmallow	23	1 Keebler Chips Deluxe Chocolate Lovers cookie	80
½ slice DiGiorno Pepperoni frozen pizza	165	2 slices Little Caesar's Pepperoni Pizza and 12 oz. Coke Classic	560
½ plain bagel (3½" diameter)	144	9 chocolate chip cookies from refrigerated dough	531
1 homemade oatmeal cookie (2⅝" diameter)	67	3½ homemade oatmeal cookies (2⅝" diameter)	235
½ slice Pillsbury Light Yellow cake (no frosting)	115	2 slices Pillsbury Light Yellow cake (no frosting)	460
½ tablespoon Jif Creamy Peanut Butter	47	1 McDonald's Sausage Patty	170
½ peanut butter sandwich (traditional PB&J made with two slices of white bread, two tablespoons of peanut butter, and two tablespoons of grape jelly)	216	1 PB&J, 12 oz. Coke, and 1 oz. potato chips (432+140+155)	727
¼ peanut butter sandwich (traditional PB&J made with two slices of white bread, two tablespoons of peanut butter, and two tablespoons of grape jelly)	108	1 PB&J sandwich	432
1 broiled boneless pork chop (Pork, Fresh, Loin, Sirloin Chops, Boneless)	177	3 pork chops (Pork, Fresh Loin, Sirloin Chops, Boneless)	620
1 slice beef bologna	88	3⅔ slices beef bologna	323

Based on a 2300 calories-per-day human diet

60-pound Dog
Requiring 890 to 950 Calories Per Day

If Your Dog Eats This ...	Number of Calories	It's Like You Eating That ...	Number of Calories
½ fried hamburger patty (50 g)	118	1 McDonald's Cheeseburger	310
¼ peanut butter sandwich (Peanut butter sandwich using Jif Reduced Fat (creamy) and Sara Lee 100% Whole Wheat bread)	82	1 slice Pizza Hut Thin 'N Crispy Pepperoni Pizza (large)	200
½ peanut butter sandwich (Peanut butter sandwich using Jif Reduced Fat, creamy, and Sara Lee 100% Whole Wheat bread)	216	1½ cups chocolate ice cream	429
½ slice Domino's Thin Crust Sausage and Pepperoni Pizza (large)	143	1 Burger King Original Whopper Junior	370
3 Pringles Original Potato Chips	28	1 Chips Ahoy Chunky Chocolate Chip Cookie	80
1 Slim Jim Original Beef Jerky Snack	43	1 1-oz. bag Rold Gold Pretzel Rods	110

Based on a 2300 calories-per-day human diet

80-pound Dog Requiring 1200 to 1500 Calories Per Day			
If Your Dog Eats This . . .	Number of Calories	It's Like You Eating That . . .	Number of Calories
1 scrambled whole egg— Grade A large	101	1 slice French toast with butter	178
½ cup mashed potatoes from flakes (made with whole milk and butter)	102	1 Twix Ice Cream Bar	170
1 cup cooked spaghetti, no sauce	220	1 Burger King Original Whopper Jr. with Cheese (low carb version)	464

Based on a 2300 calories-per-day human diet

This cycle of excess calories goes on almost unnoticed unless you are tracking your progress. Infrequent weighing combined with the Reward Rule adds up to weight gain, despite exercising and diet food. Don't focus on a specific weight, but view trends. If your pet's weight is going up over a three-month period, it's time to alter your strategy. If your dog is losing weight over a three-month period, continue with what you're doing.

Keep the 60:40 and Reward rules in the front of your mind as you approach your dog's weight loss. By understanding these concepts and recognizing these behaviors, you are much more likely to succeed.

I Didn't Bargain on the Begging!
What to Do When Your Dog Begs

When you start a weight-loss program, your dog is not going to like it. Dogs, much like their two-legged companions, don't like change. Many times dogs have received tasty treats every time they went outside for their entire life. They don't like it when they aren't rewarded with food anymore. And when dogs don't like something, they let you know it.

They do this primarily by relying on behaviors that have always worked on humans. They whine, or they stand on their back legs and dance to show you how good they are. Often, when they look at you a certain way, they get whatever they want, most notably a treat or food.

If "the look" fails, they move to Plan P: Pester. Their tactics might include whimpering and crying, pacing and pawing, or waking you in the middle of the night in an effort to get more food. Some dogs even resort to aggression in the form of destroying items or intimidating other household pets to secure more food.

This type of behavior in humans is called "hedonic hunger" and "hedonic eating." "Hedonic" is derived from the Greek word for "pleasure." The concept of hedonic hunger was first introduced by Drexel University psychologists in 2006. Hedonic eating describes how human food consumption has progressed beyond eating for energy into eating for pleasure. Our environment, emotions, and social attitudes all encourage us to eat excessively. Foods containing fat, sugar, and salt have the greatest ability to cause or encourage excessive consumption.

Hedonic Food Begging

I believe dogs experience much the same feelings toward food as we do. When dogs demonstrate excessive pleading for food, they're displaying hedonic food begging. They are begging for food they want, not need. They feel compelled to eat because of previous habit (i.e., as a reward for going potty), association (i.e., every day before the owner leaves for work they receive a treat), or as a result of changes in their neurochemistry caused by the consumption of high-sugar and high-fat foods. These dogs have real food cravings, no different than humans have, that make adhering to a diet a challenge. Instead of being able to resist the temptation of an extra scoop of ice cream or pie, dog owners must be able to withstand the withdrawal signs of hedonic eating from their dog. What you, the dog owner, are confronted with is the question of *how do I deal with the begging?*

Dogs Don't Do Division

First of all, I want to be clear that I am not against giving your dog, or yourself, treats. I am against excessive and inappropriate use of treats. If treats constitute more than 10 percent of your dog's daily calories, that's too much. I encourage you to use treats in training, but not in large amounts. As I've said to countless clients over the years, "Dogs don't do division." Dogs get the same pleasure and reward from one-third of a cookie as they do from a whole one.

> ❝ Dogs get the same pleasure and reward from one-third of a cookie as they do from a whole one. ❞

Breaking the Treat Habit

Division. If you're currently in the habit of using treats to reward your dog, start by breaking them into smaller portions. If your pet begins begging, an initial step is to simply reduce the amount of calories you're feeding in treats. This certainly doesn't achieve our ultimate goal of eliminating hedonic food begging in your dog, but it begins to change *your* behavior.

Discontinue. Use treats only if they are earned by performing some act of work. Examples of earning a treat include learning a new trick or training in a new activity. Going to the bathroom should not be viewed as work for a trained adult dog. When my daughters were toddlers, I rewarded them with all sorts of goodies during the potty-training stage. As young ladies, I do not buy them another *Magic Tree House* book when they use the commode for seven consecutive days. The same principle should be considered with adult dogs. Instead of reaching for the customary treat each time your dog does its business, try a pat on the head and verbal praise. This break from routine may be met with suspicion at first: "Where's my cookie?" they seem to be saying. Like any bad habit, it often takes weeks to months before the "new normal" resets our routine and replaces bad habits.

Substitute. Many dog owners don't have the fortitude to discontinue giving their dog treats at every occasion. So if you must give treats, try substituting a healthy alternative. Dogs often love carrots (baby or sliced), celery, asparagus, and other crunchy vegetables. Ice is another goody many dogs readily accept. Another tactic is to give kibbles of your dog's diet food as a treat. Realize that substitution is simply another Band-Aid for begging. Substitution certainly helps reduce calories, but may not do much to lessen bad behaviors.

Stick to a schedule. Feed your dog at the same time each day—for example, at 7:00 in the morning and 6:00 in the evening. Try not to deviate from these times by much. The object is to allow your dog to reliably expect when it is supposed to eat. For dogs that beg during your mealtime, try feeding your dog when you begin to eat. You should also feed your begging buddy in a separate location, preferably a different room.

As your dog becomes accustomed to an eating schedule, you may notice a decrease in in-between meal urges. Dogs need and want consistency in their lives. Hedonic food begging is a by-product of want rather than need. By removing need from the equation by offering healthy food at a consistent time of day, we help create an environment where our dog can shift away from want and the negative behaviors that accompany it. If your dog needs a between-meal snack, offer a bowl of veggies.

No means no. The most important step of training your dog not to beg is consistency with your response. If you consistently ignore the begging, your dog eventually ceases the behavior. Dogs are smart; they don't persist in a losing strategy. If one approach isn't giving them what they want, they try something else. The challenge is outlasting your dog.

In cases where your dog begs while you're eating, you may need to put your dog in its crate. The crate should be placed in a different room in another part of your house, as far away as possible from the smells and sounds of dining. If you do crate your dog, try giving it a plate of crunchy vegetables, ice treats, or an interactive toy stuffed with diet food. You want your dog occupied while you're dining.

You may have to do this for weeks to months. Your dog's behaviors may have existed since it entered your home. Just as you wouldn't expect someone to quit smoking overnight, nor should you expect your dog to suddenly stop begging. Even worse, as your dog doesn't receive food or treats anymore, the frequency and intensity of their begging often increases. Think of a person trying to stop smoking; things reminding them of cigarettes seem to pop up everywhere. These cravings are, in many ways, the same as your dog desiring food and hedonic food begging. No must mean no consistently.

Train patience. Another tip to help discourage begging is training your dog to be patient. View this step as training a dog to understand that good behavior earns something and bad behavior receives nothing. Start with one of your dog's favorite foods. Make sure your dog sees (or smells) what you have. Close your hand around the food. Most dogs will begin to nudge, paw, or beg. Don't open your hand until your dog relaxes. If your dog begins to bite or scratch you, don't say or do anything other than put the food away and repeat the exercise later. Saying "No!" or "Stop!" probably will only confuse your dog. The old rules were that they got whatever they wanted by these actions. You are trying to establish new rules of conduct.

Once your dog relaxes, give the reward and lavish praise upon them. Repeat this exercise several times a day, especially around meals. In dog training it's not the size of the reward, it's the reward itself. Hopefully this technique will help your dog learn that food and goodies are earned through calm and quiet as opposed to barking and begging.

Don't Raise Your Voice

The vocabulary of most dogs is pretty limited. Studies indicate that dogs have the approximate intelligence of a human toddler. Without debating how much your dog understands you, let's be clear on one point: our dogs do fully understand our feelings and intentions. In other words, your dog knows when you're happy or sad and also understands what you want it to do. The trouble is, not unlike a bright but petulant child, they also know our limits. Dogs are smart enough to figure out that if they beg for ten minutes, they'll get what they want. They disregard all your no's, hush's, and getaway's until they exceed that magic threshold and you give in.

When a dog doesn't respond to commands, most dog owners tend to increase their volume, as we do in human communication. He who shouts loudest wins (just watch any political roundtable if you need verification). "No" quickly escalates into *"NO!!"* I don't recommend treating your dog this way, even though I've felt like yelling at my dog before.

Dogs are primarily nonverbal communicators. They evaluate scents, body language, and expression to determine meaning. Because we don't possess the same scent-making abilities of dogs, we must focus on body language.

If your dog is begging, instead of shushing it away, maintain a strong, confident posture and simply ignore it. Don't make eye contact; don't look at the dog. Think in your mind, *I want you to stop begging and go way.* Believe it or not, your thoughts control your body. If you create the intention within your mind, your body expresses your thoughts. Your dog senses these subtle changes, which are often imperceptible to humans. At first the dog will think you're bluffing and continue with its behavior. As the dog learns you're not relying on your old bag of tricks, confusion sets in. In the dog's state of internal conflict, you have the opportunity to change its behavior. As your dog relaxes and ceases begging or barking, you acknowledge the change. Give your dog a quick glance and praise. These nonverbal and verbal signals tell your dog you liked whatever it just did.

Most dogs at this early point in training will then resume their old behavior; they're confused. You must return to your calm and confident posture and continue ignoring any begging behaviors. This back-and-forth may take weeks. Eventually your dog will give up begging. You must remain committed to breaking this cycle to succeed. This is not to say your dog will stop all forms of begging, just the all-dinner-long, every-time-I-open-the-refrigerator kind.

Why Is It So Hard to Change?

You need to overcome two key components when helping your dog lose weight: your own feelings toward obesity and weight loss, and your dog's instinct and design for energy storage. One component (ours) is psychological, and the other (our dog's) is physiological. Both are equally challenging and have different approaches for overcoming them.

When it comes to our personal resistance to change, even changes concerning our pets, we often make the critical mistake of intertwining our own beliefs with our pet's issues. We project our personal feelings, experiences, and attitudes on our pets. To change, we must first separate our personal feelings and remain as objective as possible. If we're uncomfortable with our weight, we must be careful not to allow those feelings to interfere with sound judgment and reasoning about our pet's health. Too many dog owners fail to adhere to a pet weight-loss program because of their feelings or experiences with their own attempts to lose weight. Even worse, some dog owners are overly sensitive about their personal excess weight or lack of physical fitness, and they view any comments about their pet's weight as an assault on their own.

When We Take Our Dog's Weight Personally

Several years ago I encountered just such a client. She was a young woman, probably in her late twenties or early thirties. I won't sugar-coat it; this lady was morbidly obese. She was about 5'2" and weighed at least 250 pounds. Despite the cool fall morning, she appeared red-cheeked and blotched as she walked the hundred or so feet from her car to our clinic's front door. She had come to our office seeking a second opinion about her five-year-old basset hound's lameness.

As you may have guessed, her dog was also dangerously obese. The normal weight of a basset hound is 40 to 60 pounds. Waldo tipped the scales at a whopping 86 pounds, the largest basset I've seen in almost twenty years of veterinary practice.

The veterinary technician escorted them into the exam room and began obtaining the medical history. According to the owner, Waldo's main problem was that he could barely get in and out of the car and was unable to walk up the stairs in their home. Before you scream for Captain Obvious, let me assure you that there was an underlying medical problem. Waldo suffered from osteoarthritis secondary to—you guessed it—obesity.

As I guided the conversation toward the inevitable topic of Waldo's weight, I noticed his owner becoming shifty in her seat. I sensed something was not going well, but I continued doing my job—talking about how to relieve Waldo's pain and improve his quality of life through diet, exercise, and weight loss.

And that's when it happened.

"That's all you doctors ever say, 'Lose weight, lose weight. Diet, exercise—it's all nonsense. I'm so sick of you doctors. Can't you think of anything else to say? I'm not paying for this load of bull. Get your-self a better routine and start helping people with their pets instead of just making fun of them. It must be so easy for you skinny people."

And with that, she was gone. Waldo, incidentally, didn't seem the least bit offended or upset even though we were talking about *his* weight.

Therein lies the rub. If dog owners aren't able to separate themselves from their pets, the veterinarian has almost no chance of helping the patient. I never mentioned Waldo's owner's weight, physical condition, or health. That wasn't within the scope of our conversation. Waldo's health was my only concern.

Please don't make this mistake. Your veterinarian isn't confronting you with your weight. Your veterinarian's job is to tell you how to keep your pet healthy or treat an illness. Pet owners who don't take their pet's weight personally are better able to provide exceptional care.

Your Dog: Fat Machine

The second key challenge to sustained weight loss is your dog's physiology. Dogs and humans, like most omnivores, are designed to survive long periods without food. They are able to do this by storing energy in the form of fat. Dogs and humans are exceptionally good at this.

 EYE ON THE SCIENCE

Dogs as a Model for Human Obesity

The February 2007 issue of the *American Journal of Medicine* published a study using dogs as a model for human obesity. This study, which examined the effects abdominal fat had on insulin resistance and the development of metabolic syndrome, proved that dogs experienced many of the same physiological changes humans do as a result of excess belly fat.

The reasons for this highly efficient fat-storage system are obvious. Dogs feed whenever they encounter food, dead or dying prey, or whenever they're fortunate enough to successfully hunt. They are primarily scavengers, so the ability to utilize a wide variety of foods (omnivorous) is an advantage. Because they may have the opportunity to consume a large number of calories during a single kill, specific adaptations such as a large stomach are beneficial. They need to maximize the calories they consume to sustain them during an uncertain future. The facility to store energy in the form of fat is a vital component if a dog is going to survive for days if not weeks when food may be scarce.

All of these mechanisms make a dog prone to excess weight. They make your job as chief weight-loss officer more difficult. Making matters worse, a dog's instinct basically tells them, "Eat when you get it because you don't know when you'll eat again." Today's dogs eat every day, despite what their instincts tell them. Whenever a dog owner remarks that his dog "wolfs down his food," he's really observing normal dog (or wolf) behavior. Making matters worse, modern high-fat and sugary foods and treats have hijacked your dog's brain chemistry, creating an addiction to food never before seen.

Don't despair; you still control access to the food pantry. All that is required to successfully help your pet lose weight is your commitment to provide better nutrition and a little daily exercise. Even though dogs and humans are fat machines, the on-off switch lies within each plate or bowl or food. It's up to you to turn it on or off.

12

WEIGHT-LOSS SUPPLEMENTS

Everyone is looking for an easy way to lose weight: pop a pill, drink a potion, or eat a magical food. The field of nutritional science is constantly seeking to find the next great get-fixed-quick cure. The appeal of discovering a natural remedy for disease and illness leads many scientists to pursue research into plants and to follow ancient tales of roots and herbs used by medicine men and shamans. Sometimes they find science; other times showmanship. Fortunately for us, decades of research have allowed consumers to enhance their health and the health of their pets with scientifically sound nutritional therapies. Conditions ranging from cancer to high blood pressure to depression and anxiety have all benefited from recent advancements in nutrition.

A dark side underlies this desire for all-natural remedies. Many of the purported health-benefit claims of various supplements and nutraceuticals are unfounded. At best, many of these supplements do nothing; at worst, they cause serious side effects.

The list of nutritional supplements claiming to help you or your dog lose weight is a long one. The following compilation presents some of the more common weight-loss supplements and the most recent scientific studies that support or disprove their effectiveness.

Omega-3 Fatty Acids—Fish Oils

Even if your pet doesn't need to lose weight, all humans, dogs, and cats benefit from adding omega-3 fatty acids to their diet. The omega-3 fatty acids you should use as supplements are docosahexaenoic acid (DHA) and eicosapentaenoic acid (EPA).

DHA and EPA are known as essential fatty acids. Dogs require them for life and must consume them in foods, because dogs can't manufacture essential fatty acids internally. A key problem our dogs face is that carbohydrate-based dog foods have little omega-3 fatty acids and excessive amounts of omega-6 fatty acids. Omega-6 fatty acids in high amounts or in an elevated ratio to omega-3 fatty acids in the body are known to be pro-inflammatory. The goal with omega-3 supplementation is to bring the ratio between omega-6 and omega-3 to a lower, more normal, and anti-inflammatory amount.

The ideal ratio of omega-3 fatty acids to omega-6 is thought to be 1:2 to 1:3. Many super-premium dog food diets contain an omega-3 to omega-6 ratio of 1:10.

Direct consumption of DHA and EPA from fish or algal (from algae) sources is preferred over plant sources such as flax seed. Fish oil sources of DHA and EPA are believed to have almost complete bioavailability; what a dog eats is immediately available for use. For highest absorption rates, omega-6 should not be consumed with omega-3 as they use a common enzyme for absorption.

According to a study published in the May 2004 issue of the *Journal of Veterinary Internal Medicine*, DHA and EPA seem to enhance weight loss in obese dogs. A group of obese male beagles were divided into two groups. Both groups were placed on a low-calorie diet, but one group was supplemented with tallow (beef fat) as a poor source of omega-3 fatty acid (0.2 percent) and the second group was supplemented with fish oil as an ideal omega-3 source (4.1 percent).

Both groups lost weight during the fourteen-week experiment, but the fish-oil group lost significantly more than the fat-fed dogs. In addition, total body fat and the fat-derived hormone leptin both were lower in the dogs fed fish oil.

Supplement your dog's diet with omega-3 fatty acids whether or not your pet is on a weight-loss program. The general guideline is about 30 mg per pound per day of DHA and EPA. Thus, a 20-pound dog would need about 600 mg per day of added DHA and EPA. Many dogs with heart disease, skin condition, and osteoarthritis may benefit from consuming more than 30 mg per pound per day. It is not recommended that your dog consume more than 3000 mg DHA and EPA per day unless specifically directed by your veterinarian.

Dog's weight in pounds	Suggested DHA/EPA supplementation per day in milligrams (mg)[A]
5	150–200
10	300–350
15	450–500
20	600–700
25	750–850
30	900–1000
35	1050–1150
40	1200–1300
45	1350–1450
50	1500–1600
60	1800–1900
70	2100–2200
80	2400–2500
90	2700–2800
100	3000–3100

*This chart is intended only as a guide. Consult with your veterinarian to determine the safe and appropriate dosage for your pet. Many dogs benefit from higher doses.

Not all omega-3 fatty acid supplements are created equal. Carefully review the label and determine the amount of DHA and EPA in the supplement you are using.

Omega-3 supplement	How supplied	Total omega-3 (mg)	DHA (mg)	EPA (mg)
Welactin for Dogs	Capsule	270	105	165
Welactin Canine Liquid	Liquid	1300 per teaspoon (5 ml)	525	775
Nordic Naturals Omega-3 Pet	Capsule	321	110	165
Nordic Naturals Pet Cod Liver Oil	Liquid	1000 per teaspoon	625	410
Derm Caps—for small and medium dogs	Capsule	42 mg	17	25
Derm Caps Liquid	Liquid	65mg/ml	26	39
Derm Caps ES (Extra Strength)	Capsule	126mg	50	76
Derm Caps ES Liquid	Liquid	130mg/ml	52	78
DVM 3V Caps For Large & Giant Breeds of Dogs	Capsule	1488	167	250
DVM 3V Caps For Medium Breeds of Dogs	Capsule	1100	120	180
DVM 3V Caps For Cats and Small Dogs	Capsule	670	68	103
DVM 3V Caps HP Snip Tip For Smaller Dogs and Cats	Capsule/Liquid	787.5	175	270
DVM 3V Caps HP Snip Tip For Medium To Large Dogs	Capsule/Liquid	1545.5	350	540
1-800-PetMeds Super Pure Omega 3	Capsule	1000	120	180

When selecting omega-3 fatty acid supplements, remember that supplements vary widely in terms of the amounts and ratios of DHA and EPA. For most products only about a third of the fish oil is DHA and EPA, although a "concentrated" product may contain twice or more of that amount as DHA and EPA. Thus, a fish oil claiming 1000 mg may only contain about 300 mg of DHA and EPA.

Second, the ratio of EPA to DHA will vary based on the omega-3 source. Supplements made from menhaden and other small oily fish typically have a ratio of EPA to DHA of 1.5:1, so in a capsule claiming 1 gram (1000 mg) of fish oil, typically 30 percent is EPA and DHA, thus providing your dog with 180 mg of EPA and 120 mg of DHA. Salmon oil often contains several times more DHA than EPA, and products made from algal oil contain only DHA, arguably the more important omega-3 fatty acid. If you purchase a more concentrated supplement, you are often able to give fewer capsules to your dog. Make life easier whenever possible!

You may encounter semisynthetic forms of EPA and DHA that will be labeled as "ester." These newer products claim to be as active as the natural or "triacylglycerol" forms of DHA and EPA. We do not have enough studies yet to determine if this is the case or not. One preliminary study in rats suggests that the actions of these newer products may not be the same as the naturally occurring omega-3 fatty acids. You should use natural fish oil, especially salmon products, or algae-derived omega-3.

Many fish oil supplements also contain vitamin E or other antioxidants to stabilize the oils and prevent them from becoming rancid.

If you'd prefer to add fish directly to your dog's diet, here is a list of fish rich in omega-3 fatty acids:

Anchovies	Herring
Bluefish	Lake trout
Halibut	Salmon

| Spanish mackerel | Whitefish |
| Striped sea bass | White tuna (albacore) |

I do not recommend feeding your dog (or yourself) any farm-raised fish for fear of contamination, especially from polychlorinated biphenyls (PCBs).

Flaxseed

While there are numerous health benefits of adding flax to your or your dog's diet, the reality is that flax seed or oil is not an ideal omega-3 fatty acid (DHA/EPA) supplement.

Flax seed oil contains about 45 to 60 percent of the omega-3 fatty acid alpha-linolenic acid (ALA). Other sources of ALA include canola, soy, and walnut oil. In addition, flax oil contains about 14 percent omega-6 fatty acid linoleic acid. The rest of flax oil is various monounsaturated fats. I recommend that instead of flax seed, you give your dog a fish or algal source of omega-3 fatty acids (DHA and EPA) instead of flax seed or oil.

L-Carnitine

Carnitine is another popular supplement for human weight loss. In cells, carnitine is primarily required for the transport and breakdown of fatty acids into the mitochondria (the cell's powerhouse) during energy production.

In dogs, carnitine has been shown to aid weight loss and preserve lean muscle mass, which is a critical challenge of a safe weight-loss program: how to lose fat and not muscle? For this reason, supplement carnitine in the diet of a dog on a weight-loss program.

In 1998, researchers from the Iams Company studied obese dogs (42–43 percent body fat) for nineteen weeks. These obese dogs were fed a dry, low-fat, low-fiber food with or without added L-carnitine. The dogs were given either 50 mg/kg or 100 mg/kg carnitine added into the diet. Dogs that ate the diet plus carnitine lost more weight compared to the food-only group. The study also found that the dogs given L-carnitine had higher lean muscle mass and lower body fat.

A 1999 study conducted by Hill's Pet Nutrition also found carnitine to be helpful in pet weight loss. These dogs were given carnitine added to their food for six months while being fed a low-fat, high-fiber diet. The dogs given carnitine lost more weight and had more lean muscle mass and less body fat than the dogs not receiving the supplement.

Natural sources of carnitine include meat, fish, and poultry. In general, higher carnitine levels are found in redder meats. Whey protein also contains a small amount of carnitine.

I recommend administering L-carnitine for weight loss in dogs. The general recommended dosage range for L-carnitine in dogs is 10 to 70 mg/pound three times a day. I typically begin my smaller patients, those weighing less than 20 pounds, on 250 mg twice daily, and dogs 20 to 40 pounds on 500 mg twice daily. Higher doses or more frequent administration may be used in certain situations. Carnitine is typically available in 250 mg and 500 mg capsules.

Weight in pounds	Suggested carnitine starting dosage as a weight-loss supplement
0–20	250 mg every 12 hours
20–60	500 mg every 12 hours
60–80	1000 mg every 12 hours
80+	1000 mg every 8 hours

Diacylglycerol

The past few years have seen an emergence of novel weight-loss products. One of the more interesting and promising supplements is an ingredient of many oils used in foods, diacylglycerol (DAG). DAG seems to have effects on fat and glucose metabolism. Research indicates that it may lower blood fat levels (triglycerides), decrease blood fat levels after eating, increase metabolism, reduce body fat, and enhance weight loss.

With the approval of DAG for use in foods in the United States, many companies are beginning to replace their traditional oil with DAG. But does it help dogs lose weight? Early studies seem to indicate so.

A June 2006 study in the *Journal of Animal Physiology and Animal Nutrition* examined dogs fed a diet made with diacylglycerol oil. The researchers focused on using only diacylglycerol without reducing calories. Diacylglycerol oil was simply substituted for triacylglycerol oil.

Researchers fed overweight beagles with either a DAG or traditional triacylglycerol oil diet for six weeks. The diets had the same nutrient profile otherwise. Dogs fed the diacylglycerol diet showed a statistically significant reduction in body weight, averaging a 2.3 percent reduction in six weeks, while the triacylglycerol-diet dogs maintained their starting obese weights. Even more impressive was the finding that the diacylglycerol group also showed a reduction in body fat content, blood fats (serum triglyceride), and total cholesterol—all without reducing calories. Another study published in the 2006 *Journal of Nutrition* substantiated these findings.

These studies indicate that if dog food manufactures would develop a food using diacylglycerol, it may help control weight and reduce blood fat levels without requiring a decrease in calories. Patents for using diacylglycerol in pet foods have already been filed. I hope we will soon have dog foods made with diacylglycerol oil available for use. Diacylglycerol oil is currently manufactured under the name Enova Oil. You can use it in your own cooking and for your dog's home-cooked meals whenever oil is needed.

If you choose to add DAG to your dog's current diet, you'll need to adjust the amount of calories you feed your dog. Like many oils, DAG is calorically dense. One tablespoon of Enova Oil contains 120 calories, all of them from fat. Because DAG is a fat source with significant calories, I do not recommend simply pouring it over your dog's food.

Conjugated Linoleic Acid (CLA)

Conjugated linoleic acid (CLA) is a fatty acid found primarily in meat dairy products and vegetable oils. CLA has long been associated with a wide variety of health benefits, including weight loss.

Unfortunately, few scientific studies support the weight-loss claim in dogs. In a 2004 *Federation of American Societies for Experimental Biology Journal* study, researchers fed some dogs a high-protein, low-carbohydrate diet with and without added CLA and other dogs a control diet with and without CLA. Dogs fed CLA showed no additional weight loss compared to dogs not given CLA.

Another study published in the summer 2006 issue of *Veterinary Therapeutics* evaluated dogs fed a high-fiber diet with and without added CLA. Dogs on the diet plus CLA did not lose any more weight than the dogs fed a high-fiber diet alone.

My recommendation is to use CLA only under your veterinarian's supervision. Not enough consistent scientific studies endorse its widespread use as a weight-loss supplement. There may be other reasons to give your dog CLA, and future studies may validate it as an appropriate part of a weight-loss strategy. Some dogs may experience temporary gastrointestinal upset (vomiting and diarrhea) when taking CLA.

Chromium

Chromium is an essential dietary trace mineral involved in carbohydrate and lipid metabolism. Research in the past decade has focused on chromium as an aid in glucose control, especially in diabetic patients. In dogs, chromium has been used with mixed results as an aid in the treatment of diabetes and as a weight-loss supplement.

A June 2008 *Journal of Veterinary Internal Medicine* study concluded that administering chromium to diabetic dogs had no effect on
average body weight, daily insulin dosage, daily caloric intake, ten-
hour mean blood glucose concentration, blood-glycated hemoglobin
concentration, and serum fructosamine concentration. Several other
studies failed to show a benefit to weight loss. Further, some studies
have shown high doses of chromium picolinate may damage DNA. If
you choose to supplement chromium in your dog's diet, do so under
your veterinarian's close supervision and use low doses.

DHEA

The scientific literature is full of contradicting studies on dehydroepiandrosterone (DHEA) in dogs. DHEA is one of the body's most
prevalent steroids, involved in the production of several sex hormones,
including testosterone and the estrogens estrone and estradiol. In dogs,
its weight-loss effect is marred by the fact that the high doses needed
to promote lean body mass may cause adverse side effects from the
excess production of sex hormones.

A January 1998 *Journal of Obesity Research* study evaluated the
addition of DHEA to a low-fat, high-fiber diet. The University of
Wisconsin researchers found that dogs given DHEA lost more weight
faster than placebo-treated dogs. They concluded that DHEA in combination with a low-calorie diet caused a faster rate of weight loss than
reducing calories alone. In addition, the study found that DHEA low-
ered cholesterol, especially LDL or "bad" cholesterol. Critics later
were concerned that the high doses used in the study may cause the
production of excess sex hormones.

Supplementing DHEA at low doses, 5 to 50 mg per day, may provide your dog some weight-loss benefit with little risk. 7-oxo-DHEA
may be a safer alternative to DHEA for weight loss in dogs. The exact
dosage for 7-oxo-DHEA has not been established for dogs, although it

appears to be safe, even at high levels. There are many reasons to supplement DHEA in your dog's diet, especially with regards to reducing the stress hormone cortisol. Talk to your veterinarian before giving your dog DHEA.

Weight-Loss Supplements That Don't Add Up: Save Your Money and Skip Them

For a number of supplements, the science is simply lacking, and I cannot recommend them as part of a dog's weight-loss program.

Pyruvate

In the mid- to late 1990s, the weight-loss world found pyruvate, which was discovered to be a key component in the cell's production of energy. The theory was that adding pyruvate to the diet would increase metabolism and help break down fat, thereby aiding in weight loss.

Pyruvate has been shown to assist in weight loss in humans and rats, but not in dogs. If you choose to give pyruvate to your dog, the current recommendation is to use the human dose of 2 grams per day. Be sure to read the label of any pyruvate supplement carefully. Many labels are difficult to understand unless you look at the guaranteed analysis. Most human supplements contain 2 grams per capsule.

Starch Blockers

Imagine a product that would block your body's conversion of carbohydrates to sugar and fat. You could eat all the jelly doughnuts you desired, pop a starch blocker, and never gain an ounce. This claim is the promise of the so-called starch blockers, or amylase inhibitors.

Manufacturers of starch blockers assert that they block a key enzyme in the utilization of carbohydrates: alpha amylase. The general theory is that by blocking this enzyme, the body is prevented from breaking down the starch found in foods like potatoes, pasta, muffins, and bread.

If the body doesn't break down starch, you wouldn't acquire extra calories from the carbs you consume. Where's that jelly doughnut?

Unfortunately, scientific studies don't support the claims. The most recent study, published in the July/August 2007 issue of *Alternative Therapies*, found no significant weight loss in the group given a white bean extract (a starch blocker) in addition to the multiple components of diet, exercise, and behavior during a four-week study. Earlier studies published in a 1982 issue of the *New England Journal of Medicine* and a 1983 issue of *Science* also found no advantage to taking a starch blocker. No similar studies exist for overweight dogs.

As appealing as the idea of a starch blocker is, I do not use them in my weight-loss patients at this time. There does not appear to be any significant health risk in using a starch blocker in dogs, although vomiting, diarrhea, and loose stools may be associated with taking a starch blocker.

Chitosan

Chitosan is a compound made from the shells of crustaceans such as shrimp, crab, and other shellfish. Manufacturers suggest that chitosan or chitin binds with fat molecules within the intestine, thereby preventing fat absorption. At this time there have been no studies conducted to see if chitosan aids dogs with weight loss. I do not recommend the use of chitosan or chitin as a weight-loss supplement.

Vitamin A

Supplementing your dog's diet with Vitamin A is unlikely to be necessary if you are feeding a nutritious, well-balanced diet. No studies of dogs support the use of Vitamin A as an aid in weight loss.

Soy Protein and Flaxseed

Many positive benefits can result from feeding your dog soy protein and flaxseed, none of which are proven to involve weight loss. I support and encourage the use of soy protein in dogs but until more scientific studies are conducted, I am hesitant to make a weight loss claim for soy protein and flaxseed with lignans.

Hydroxycitric Acid

The source of hydroxycitric acid, the Indian tropical fruit tamarind (*Garcinia cambogia*), is reported to help fight excess weight and promote health. It is claimed to increase the metabolism of fats. Human and rat studies have thus far shown mixed results. It appears to be safe, but no studies in dogs have been performed at this time. I do not recommend using hydroxycitric acid as a weight-loss supplement in dogs because of the current lack of scientific and safety studies. It is marketed as tamarind, Garcinia, Malabar, HCA, and HA.

Ephedra and Caffeine Compounds

Ephedra sinica (*Ma huang* in Chinese) is a shrub native to China and Mongolia. Ephedra is also known as sea ephedrine, ephedra alkaloids, sea grape, yellow horse, yellow astringent, joint fir, squaw tea, Mormon tea, popotillo, and teamster's tea. Ephedra has not been evaluated by the FDA for safety, effectiveness, or purity. Because ephedra has been reported to cause serious, even fatal, side effects such as heart attack, stroke, irregular heartbeats, and sudden death in people, the FDA has recommended that ephedra not be taken.

Ephedra is often combined with a caffeine source as a weight-loss supplement. Green tea, guarana, and yerba maté are often found in ephedra products. Additionally, stimulants such as phenethylamine (PEA) may be added.

Dogs appear to be very sensitive to many stimulants and should not be given products containing them. I do not recommend the use of ephedra or caffeine-containing products for weight loss in dogs due to serious concerns for safety.

Glucomannan, Psyllium, and Guar Gum

Many weight-loss supplements contain various sources of soluble fiber, which, in theory, could promote weight loss by absorbing water in the gut, resulting in increased satiety and reduced food consumption. Soluble fiber has also been reported to aid in the treatment of diabetes and to lower blood fats.

Glucomannan (*Amorphophallus konjac*), psyllium, and guar gum (derived from *Cyamopsis tetragonolobus*, the Indian cluster bean) are all commonly available sources of soluble fiber.

While these products appear safe, no studies in dogs have evaluated their usage as a weight-loss supplement. Studies in humans have shown little benefit from these compounds in weight loss. Guar gum in particular has been carefully investigated and no weight-loss benefits were found.

I do not recommend using these substances as a weight-loss supplement in dogs.

Spirulina

Spirulina, also known as blue-green algae or cyanobacteria, has been reported to suppress appetite in humans. Spirulina contains phenylalanine, an essential amino acid found in the breast milk of mammals. Because it is a direct precursor to phenylethylamine, a commonly used dietary supplement, phenylalanine is said to inhibit appetite.

In 1981, the FDA declared Spirulina ineffective for weight loss in humans. I do not recommend the use of Spirulina for weight loss in dogs. However, giving your dog a microalgae supplement can have other nutritional benefits, especially in older or ill pets.

Vitamin B$_5$

Vitamin B5 or pantothenic acid has been suggested as a weight-loss supplement in people. In a 1995 article in *Medical Hypotheses*, the researcher proposed a technique for weight loss that involved fasting and supplementing with high doses of Vitamin B5. While this approach theoretically may work, no clinical trials to date have taken place.

I recommend giving your dog a daily B-vitamin supplement. There is no scientific or clinical evidence that B vitamins aid in weight loss, though.

Dandelion and Cascara

Dandelion extract (*Taraxacum officinale*) appears to have diuretic or water-losing properties. Cascara (*Rhamnus purshiana*) acts a laxative, according to the *Physician's Desk Reference for Herbal Medicines*. Cascara is also known as Cascara buckthorn, bearberry, chittam, or chitticum.

Long-term use of these supplements could result in serious consequences, including dehydration and electrolyte imbalances.

I do not recommend the use of dandelion extract or cascara as a weight-loss agent in dogs. No studies on its efficacy or safety in dogs have yet been conducted.

Ginseng

Ginseng (*Panax ginseng*) is a well-known Chinese herb. Its proponents claim that ginseng reduces stress, acts as an aphrodisiac and stimulant, and can be used to treat type 2 diabetes and sexual dysfunction in men. Newer claims that ginseng may help reduce appetite have led to its inclusion in several weight-loss products.

Not many studies have evaluated ginseng in dogs. An August 2007 study published in the *Journal of Veterinary Pharmacology and Therapeutics* evaluated the effect a product containing ginseng and brewer's yeast, Gerivet, had as a stimulant on older dogs. The researchers found that the dogs receiving ginseng and brewer's yeast had owner-reported improvements in the dog's general status. Ginseng was thought to be responsible for the mental improvements and brewer's yeast the physical benefits. There were no reported safety issues.

There has been no ginseng weight-loss study performed on dogs at this time. I do recommend the use of ginseng as a general supplement in older dogs experiencing mental or physical decline.

Probiotics

Suddenly, probiotics are in everything we eat. They're also coming to a dog food near you, if they haven't already. Probiotics promise many health benefits—some real, others unfounded—and should be considered as part of a dog's healthy diet.

What Are Probiotics?

The UN Food and Agriculture Organization and the World Health Organization officially defined the term "probiotics" in 2001 as "live microorganisms which when administered in adequate amounts confer a health benefit on the host." In other words, a bacterium or product containing bacteria is considered a probiotic if the bacteria have been shown to be alive at time of use and in sufficient quantity to confer a physiologic health benefit.

You should be aware of two other terms. *Prebiotics* are dietary substances that serve as food for the probiotic bacteria. These substances feed the bacteria either in a probiotic or the intestinal tract. Common prebiotics include complex sugars such as inulin, oligofructose, and lactulose and other fructo-oligosaccharides. Fructo-oligosaccharides are carbohydrates found in fruit. "Fructo" means "fruit," and an oligosaccharide is a type of carbohydrate. Natural sources of prebiotics for dogs include oatmeal, wheat, barley, legumes, bananas, berries, leafy greens, and leeks. While the words "prebiotics" and "probiotics" are very similar, they are completely different things. Prebiotics feed bacteria; probiotics *are* bacteria.

"Synbiotic" is another term you may see on some food or supplement labels. Some probiotic-infused dairy products have prebiotics added to help the friendly microbes survive in the intestinal tract. Synbiotics are foods for the probiotics (bacteria) in a supplement, and prebiotics are food for the bacteria already living in the intestine. You can see how easy it is to confuse these terms—and marketers take full advantage of that. Remember that products containing ingredients such as berries or leeks can be labeled as "containing prebiotics." To the uneducated eye, that looks awfully similar to "probiotics."

How Do Probiotics Work?

The question of how probiotics confer health benefits has been one of intense investigation. The normal canine gastrointestinal tract contains thousands of different species and subspecies of bacteria, referred to as the *intestinal flora*. When the normal balance of these bacteria is altered by sickness or antibiotics, many dogs develop diarrhea. Probiotics work by recolonizing or inoculating the small intestine with helpful bacteria that may have been reduced. These bacteria help reestablish the normal bacterial balance in the intestine by blocking problem-causing bacteria. They may also produce substances that inhibit harmful bacteria, compete for nutrients with them, and stimulate the body's own immune system.

Why Does Your Dog Need Probiotics?

Many factors alter your dog's normal healthy intestinal microflora. Some of the common causes of changes in the gut bacteria are:

Aging	Illness
Anesthetic agents	Stress
Anthelmetics (Dewormers)	Suboptimal diet
Antibiotics	

The concept of treatment with probiotics comes from a belief that modern humans do not consume or replenish the beneficial microbes in their bodies and that they can do so by taking probiotics. This belief is now applied to dogs. But simply eating more bacteria does not in itself guarantee good health. Most probiotic products available for humans and dogs are foods containing *Lactobacillus* or *Bifidobacteria,* bacteria that don't cause infection and are common in a healthy gut and vagina. These bacteria have been used for more than a century as health supplements.

Do Probiotics Work?

Recent studies are beginning to prove through advanced genetic testing that probiotics do indeed benefit our health and the health of many animals. A 2008 study published in *Molecular Systems Biology* proved that probiotics given to laboratory mice produced genetic changes across several metabolic pathways. The researchers concluded that probiotic supplementation may play a role in an animal's overall metabolic health. We are beginning to see generations of anecdotal reports of the health benefits of probiotics proven through advanced laboratory testing methods.

When Should I Give Probiotics?

There is considerable debate over the benefit of giving your dog (or yourself) probiotics on a routine basis. I recommend you inoculate your healthy dog with probiotics monthly with a proven pet-specific probiotic. I make this suggestion based on the fact that we live in an environment that may be stressful or polluted, most dogs (and people) do not eat an ideal diet, and our pets are exposed to many medications and treatments that constantly affect the intestinal microflora. I also advise that less healthy or more stressed (mentally or physically) dogs may benefit from more frequent inoculations with probiotics, perhaps weekly.

Overweight dogs may benefit greatly from probiotic usage, and I typically recommend weekly treatment with a canine-specific probiotic until the desired weight is achieved. There is no clear consensus on if, when, and how you should use probiotics in dogs. Until conclusive studies in dogs are performed, these recommendations must be based on studies conducted primarily in mice and humans. Even adding non-fat plain yogurt to the diet has been shown to help some people.

I also recommend giving your dog probiotics in the following situations:

- Mild to moderate acute idiopathic diarrhea
- Anticipated stress
- Extended travel or boarding
- Postanesthesia diarrhea
- Postantibiotic diarrhea
- Inflammatory bowel disease
- Seasonal allergies
- Urinary tract infections

How Do I Choose a Probiotic?

An exciting array of probiotics is available for dogs. Unfortunately, neither the FDA nor any other federal or state agency routinely tests probiotics for quality prior to sale. However, consider the following when selecting a probiotic for your dog:

- Look for a product containing at least 1 billion organisms.
- The product should contain only the bacteria it claims on the label. In a recent Consumer Lab study, one probiotic product for dogs was found to contain only mold.
- Several types of bacteria, including *Lactobacillus bulgaricus* and *Streptococcus thermophilus*, as well as *Leuconostoc* and *Lactococcus* species, cannot survive as they pass through stomach acid and into the small intestine. The product should contain either bacteria proven to survive passage through the stomach, or it should be enteric coated if not. Products in tablets and capsules should be proven to disintegrate in the small intestine and not pass undigested in the stool.

I recommend consulting a third-party supplement review source such as Consumer Lab (www.ConsumerLab.com) when purchasing a probiotic or other supplement.

Choosing Supplements for Your Dog

One of the most frequent questions dog owners ask is, "Which brand of supplement should I give my dog?" Unfortunately, the answer boils down to your trust in the company and the little, if any, oversight to which the companies may subject themselves. Neither the FDA, USDA, nor AAFCO regulates, inspects, or oversees nutritional supplements or nutraceuticals in the United States. As long as a supplement doesn't cause reported illness or make label claims that are unsubstantiated, it can be sold, regardless of whether it works or even contains what the label says. A supplement could be made from sawdust, and as long as it didn't harm anyone or any animal or claim a druglike action, it can be sold, no questions asked. That's a pretty scary thought and one of the reasons so many physicians and veterinarians are reluctant to recommend nutritional supplements. Physicians and veterinarians have no assurances that the patient would actually receive the ingredient recommended.

Herbal supplements are, however, regulated by the FDA, which requires the producers to follow good manufacturing practices: sanitary production conditions, proper identification of active ingredients, and assuring that the product is not contaminated and is fit for consumption. Unfortunately, the FDA's ability to strictly monitor and inspect supplement manufacturers may be inadequate to guarantee safety. Sadly, veterinary supplements are arguably even less closely monitored by the FDA than human products. Buying supplements for your dog is truly a case of caveat emptor.

Before starting your dog on a nutritional supplement, ask your veterinarian for specific recommendations and investigate the manufacturer.

As the demand for pet supplements has grown, companies with less-than-stellar histories have begun manufacturing products for veterinary use. Studies have shown that nutraceuticals are commonly mislabeled and may contain impurities, including heavy metals, toxins, bacteria, and molds. Many supplements contain variable quantities of active ingredients, while others may fail to dissolve at all and pass undigested.

Here are some general guidelines to use when choosing a supplement for your dog:

Look for the USP seal. The United States Pharmacopeia (USP) is the authority for all prescription and over-the-counter (OTC) medicines and other health-care products manufactured or sold in the United States. This nongovernmental organization's duty is to oversee products not regulated by the FDA. Companies do not have to have their products USP-verified to be sold. I recommend using USP-verified products whenever possible. Additional information about the USP verification process is available at www.usp.org/audiences/veterinary.

USP-verified Dietary Supplements carry this seal on their label.

If only certain ingredients have been USP-verified, you will find this seal.

Examine the expiration date and lot number. If these are missing from the label, do not purchase the supplement.

Look for the NADA seal. If a supplement claims a medical benefit on the label, there should be a New Animal Drug Application

(NADA) number accompanying the product. While required by law, manufacturers often ignore it. An NADA seal typically suggests higher quality because the manufacturer is abiding by FDA regulations for drug manufacture.

Read the ingredient list. All ingredients should be clearly listed in order of ingredient weight. In other words, just as with dog foods, keep the label should begin with the ingredient that is greatest in weight and continue in descending order.

Read the instructions for use. Does the supplement contain easy-to-understand dosing instructions? If not, the company may not have determined a safe and appropriate dosage.

Visit ConsumerLab.com. This website helps you search for supplements that independently verified studies, medical journal publications, and clinical studies have investigated.

Check for clinical studies. The best supplements have clinical studies backing up their health claims. Look for randomized, double-blind, placebo-controlled studies, often abbreviated RCT for "randomized clinical trial." Not every supplement has RCT data, but if it's available, choosing a supplement for use becomes much easier.

Beware of testimonials. "It's amazing!" means nothing, unless the statement comes from a respected source. "Anne M. with Boomer from Nebraska" is not such a resource, despite her incredible claims.

Consider what you're getting for the money. Less expensive compounds are more likely to be of inferior quality. Several studies of glucosamine sulfate/chondroitin supplements have shown that the cheapest supplements are often the lowest quality. Unfortunately, the most expensive ones are not always the best. In general, avoid rock-bottom-priced supplements. They're cheap for a reason, and it may not be a good one. Do your homework to get what you pay for.

Look for NASC membership. The National Animal Supplement Council (NASC) is an industry group that works closely with the FDA. The NASC has established strict quality-control and adverse-event recording guidelines for member companies. Supplements made by NASC-member companies are likely to have better-quality products. See the www.NASC.cc website for more information.

Website Resources for Nutritional Supplements

Consumer Lab	www.consumerlab.com
National Animal Supplement Council	www.nasc.cc
Natural Medicines Comprehensive Database	www.naturaldatabase.com
Natural Standard	www.naturalstandard.com
American Botanical Council	www.herbalgram.org
Nutrition Business Journal	www.nutritionbusinessjournal.com
National Center for Complementary and Alternative Medicine (NCCAM), a component of the National Institutes of Health	www.nccam.nih.gov
USDA Food and Nutrition Center, Dietary Supplements	www.nal.usda.gov/fnic
United States Pharmacopeia (USP)	www.usp.org

The Doggie Diet Pill

On January 5, 2007, the FDA approved the first weight-loss drug for dogs, Pfizer's Slentrol (dirlotapide). This drug works by reducing appetite and decreasing fat absorption. In clinical trials, almost 98 percent of dogs receiving Slentrol lost some weight during the four-month study. Reported side effects have been mild to date, consisting mainly of vomiting and loose stools.

Based on this information, you're probably wondering why there's a need for this book. It could be condensed to a single prescription pad page. Give your dog the pill; dog loses weight. End of story.

It's not quite that simple. Most dogs begin regaining weight within a couple of days of discontinuing Slentrol, because the drug suppresses the appetite, not the owner's willingness to feed his dog inappropriately. In Pfizer's own studies, they concluded that "when the drug is stopped, food intake increases." That's to be expected, except the post-Slentrol food intake was higher than for the control dogs. In fact, the dogs ate almost twice as much food per day in weeks seventeen and eighteen as they did in the sixteen weeks while on Slentrol.

This isn't a knock on Slentrol; it's a knock on the dogs' owners.

If my canine patient were making the decision to overeat and couldn't stop, I'd understand using a drug to change the way the brain handles the appetite. Instead, dog owners create this behavior and then look for an easy way to stop it. Slentrol works primarily because dogs stop showing interest in food.

If we choose to share our lives with dogs, an important part of our responsibility is to serve as stewards of good health. We need to make good choices in feeding our dogs a wholesome, balanced, and appropriate diet. If there were a drug to alter a dog owner's constant need to give her dog treats, I would wholeheartedly endorse it. I have a harder time recommending a drug that affects the innocent bystander.

When to Use a Weight-Loss Drug

Medications such as Slentrol do have a place in the war on obesity. I typically recommend using drugs to facilitate weight loss in morbidly obese dogs as a behavior-transition tool with unmotivated owners or in dogs obsessed with eating. I am careful to counsel them that the real benefit of Slentrol is to give the owners an opportunity to change the way they view and use food in their dogs' lives. When the dog reaches its ideal weight and we stop Slentrol, the previous eating behaviors will

likely return. What must change is the owner's impulse to offer goodies throughout the day or slip the dog a sausage at breakfast. If the
owner fails to change his behavior, the dog's weight will return quickly.
Yet if you are the owner of an extremely obese dog, you should consider Slentrol as part of your weight-loss strategy. I believe in keeping
all available options open when treating my patients. Slentrol has been
shown to be safe and effective since its release and needs to be a part
of any veterinarian's arsenal of potential treatments.

New Drugs on the Horizon?

Because the market for anti-obesity drugs in the United States is
estimated to be over $200 million annually, other drug companies are
eager to get in on the action. In September 2009, Stirling Products
Limited announced promising results from phase-one clinical trials of
its dog weight-loss drug, R-salbutamol. Salbutamol is an example of an
older drug being used in a new way; it has been used for years to treat
asthma in humans. The trials found dogs lost an average of nearly 3
percent of their body weight per week while on the drug with few
reported side effects. While it is early in the approval process, salbutamol may be the next entry into this financially lucrative market.
Additional weight-loss drugs for dogs are likely to be introduced in the
near future as well. Mitrapide, liraglutide and others fill the rumor
mill. Dog owners should carefully evaluate the need for medicinal
treatment of a problem that can be successfully—and safely—treated
without prescription drugs.

A Final Word of Caution

A further concern about weight-loss drugs in dogs is the fact that
we can't accurately assess a drug's impact on a dog's behavior unless it
is profoundly obvious. How do you know if your dog is depressed if
he can't tell you? Mood swings, depression, and suicidal thoughts have
long been associated with many drugs that suppress appetite in humans.

How do you determine if a dog experiences similar negative feelings? Serious scientists will scoff at such notions, but as someone who has spent his entire life living with and caring for animals, I am convinced they have distinct feelings and thoughts. No one can prove or disprove what animals think. For me, I think it would be intellectually negligent to assume that "there's nothing going on up there in the minds of dogs." The sad truth is we don't know and we often can't tell if psychoactive medications affect our dogs in undesirable ways. Until more is known, I'll continue to be cautious when it comes to prescribing certain drugs to my patients.

13

WHEN OBESITY GOES UNCHECKED:
The Consequences of Excess Weight

Many dog owners view their pet's excess weight as no big deal. Sure, they know there could be consequences, but they've owned dogs their entire lives and never had a problem. While dogs in the past didn't seem to have as many serious medical problems, it probably isn't because they were lucky or the dogs were hardier or we took better care of them. The most likely reason is that they had shorter life expectancies. While hard data is difficult to come by, in general terms the life expectancy of dogs in the 1960s was around ten to twelve years. By 2000, that age had been extended to thirteen to fifteen years for most breeds. Today's small indoor dogs can expect to live fifteen to seventeen years or longer if they maintain a healthy lifestyle.

Shorter Life Expectancy

Obesity kills. As mentioned at the outset of this book, we're raising the first generation of dogs that likely won't live as long as their parents. But this book has given some simple solutions that begin with changing your dog's diet.

Less is more when it comes to living longer. Studies show the impact that eating less has on nearly everything in the food chain: from worms to rats, dogs, monkeys, and humans. Eating fewer calories means a longer life. But remember, caloric restriction does not mean starvation. Most studies look at reducing calories by 25 percent or about 100 calories per day for a medium-sized dog. That's the equivalent of about one-quarter to one-third of a cup of normal dog food. A little less food equals a lot more living.

 EYE ON THE SCIENCE

Calorie Restriction and Increased Life Span

The link between calorie restriction and increased life span started in 1934 at Cornell University when Dr. Clive McCay, a professor of animal husbandry, observed that laboratory rats placed on a severely reduced-calorie diet while simultaneously maintaining essential nutrient levels had life spans up to twice as long as normal lab rats.

Fifty years later, Dr. Roy Walford would popularize the theory of caloric restriction and life extension. In his best-selling book *The Retardation of Aging and Disease by Dietary Restriction*, Walford proved that reducing calories in mice increased their life span, decreased cancer rates, and improved immune function. Subsequent studies would validate his findings in numerous species of animals. He would go on to author seven books on the benefits of a low-calorie lifestyle.

The landmark study on caloric restriction in dogs was published in the May 1, 2002, issue of the *Journal of the American Veterinary Medical Association*. Forty-eight Labrador retrievers from seven litters (bred from seven females and two male mates) were studied for their entire life, about fifteen years, to determine the effects reducing their caloric intake by 25 percent had on longevity, disease incidence, and other age-related changes. The dogs were divided in half; the control group ate the number of calories necessary to maintain a normal weight, while their study counterpart received 25 percent less food. The results were stunning.

The median life span of dogs (the age when half of the dogs were deceased) in the control group fed the normal amount of calories was 11.2 years. The restricted-calorie group lived a median 13 years. *That's almost two years of extra life.* But the story didn't stop there. Not only did the dogs fed less calories live longer, they had fewer chronic diseases that affected them later in life such as arthritis. They not only lived longer; they had a better quality of life.

In the January 15, 2005, *Journal of the American Veterinary Medical Association,* the researchers elaborated on their findings. They revealed that nine of the original twenty-four calorie-restricted dogs were still living after *all* of the control dogs had died. Think about that for a moment: almost a third of the dogs fed 25 percent fewer calories were still living and having fewer medical problems after all of the dogs fed a "normal" amount of calories were dead. In fact, half of the low-calorie dogs were living at age thirteen compared to only 4 percent of the control dogs. Even moderately overweight dogs were less likely to live longer than 12 years according to a 2005 *Veterinary Clinics of North America* published report. Think about that the next time you're measuring your dog's food.

Osteoarthritis

Even if dogs live longer, if they're unable to walk and run, play, and live normally, is that an improvement? Arthritis is one of the most common reasons older dogs have a poor quality of life and are ultimately euthanized. Most cases of osteoarthritis can be avoided, given that fat is more harmful to our joints than we ever dreamed.

There are several forms of arthritis in dogs. The two most common are osteoarthritis (OA) and rheumatoid arthritis (RA). Osteoarthritis is also called degenerative joint disease (DJD) or degenerative arthritis and refers to the condition of joint degradation. Rheumatoid arthritis is a disease process caused by the immune system that, for unknown reasons, attacks and damages the joints.

When most people say "arthritis," they are referring to osteoarthritis. According to figures published in a December 2008 *American Journal of Veterinary Research* study, 20 percent of middle-aged dogs and 90 percent of older dogs were thought to have some degree of osteoarthritis. This malady is widely thought to be one of the leading causes for veterinary visits in North America.

Most of us view the relationship with being overweight and arthritis as follows: when you're overweight, more force is placed on the joints, resulting in injury and damage to the bones in the joint leading to osteoarthritis. In simplest terms, you overload your joints, the cartilage breaks down, and voila, arthritis. While that remains true, recent research indicates that the reasons obese individuals develop arthritis are more insidious.

As you now know, fat is a very active tissue. Far from being an inert lump, fat is a hormone factory, pumping out dozens of hormones and sometimes dangerous chemicals. These chemical hormones are being closely tested for their actions and their damaging effects on health.

EYE ON THE SCIENCE

Active Fat

In the December 1994 issue of *Nature*, Rockefeller University's Jeffrey M. Friedman published a landmark paper on obesity and changed how we view fat tissue. He identified a gene he cleverly called *obese (ob)* and the subit produced leptin, after the Greek word for thin, *leptos*. While Freidman's breakthrough didn't explain the link between obesity and arthritis, it did prove there was much more going on in fat than previously thought.

Leptin is primarily produced by white adipose tissue, and the more fat a dog or person has, the more leptin is circulating. When leptin was first discovered, scientists thought it would be the silver bullet to slay obesity. Because leptin decreases food intake and increases energy consumption, researchers thought they'd simply bottle it up, give it to dogs or people, and presto, instant no-effort weight loss. The media went into a frenzy. Headlines proclaimed the "end of fat" and "miracle obesity cure." Doctors puffed their chest on television screens and proclaimed science had triumphed over one of nature's cruelest tricks. Revelers in 1995 omitted dieting and exercise from their New Year's resolutions because a magic pill was on its way.

Imagine everyone's dismay when scientists later discovered that obese people had loads of leptin in their blood. Taking more of it wasn't going to cause weight loss.

The breakthrough in understanding the devastating effects of fat gained momentum with the detection of a group of hormones now called *adipokines*, *adipocytokines*, or *cytokines*. These previously unknown chemicals secreted by fat signal other cells and affect the body in a multitude of ways. Many adipokines are currently recognized in humans and laboratory mice. Leptin, adiponectin, resistin, visfatin, retinol-binding protein, and tumor necrosis factor-alpha (TNF-alpha) are just a few of the memorable names of these chemicals.

The key adipokines involved in osteoarthritis are thought to be adiponectin and leptin. Other fat-derived compounds that contribute to the development of osteoarthritis in dogs are TNF-alpha, adipose angiotensinogen (AGT), and interleukin-1 beta (IL-1 beta). In a nutshell, these compounds cause inflammation throughout the body, including the joints.

Table 1.1. Substances That Fat Produces: Their Functions and Consequences

Substance Produced by Fat Tissue	Basic Function	Potential Consequences
LEPTIN	Regulates appetite	→ Low body fat and low leptin levels cause increased appetite → High body fat and high leptin levels suppress appetite
	Biomarker of fat	Increasing obesity causes high blood leptin levels

	Pro-inflammatory substance	May cause or worsen osteoarthritis
		→ Associated with
		  ✓ Insulin resistance
		  ✓ Rheumatoid arthritis
		  ✓ Osteoarthritis
		  ✓ Hepatitis
		  ✓ Intestinal inflammation

RESISTIN	→ Produced in fat and immune cells of dogs
	→ Named because it is associated with "resistance" to insulin
		→ May lead to insulin resistance
		→ Increases liver glucose secretion despite high insulin levels
		→ Causes inflammation
		→ Associated with
		  ✓ Atherosclerosis
		  ✓ Obesity
		  ✓ Chronic kidney disease
		→ May be associated with
		  ✓ Type 2 diabetes
		  ✓ Arthritis

ADIPONECTIN	→ Involved in the control of glucose and fatty-acid metabolism	→ Improves insulin sensitivity
		→ Risk factor for metabolic syndrome in humans
		→ Causes inflammation
		→ Associated with
		  ✓ Atherosclerosis
		  ✓ Obesity
		  ✓ Rheumatoid arthritis
		  ✓ Osteoarthritis

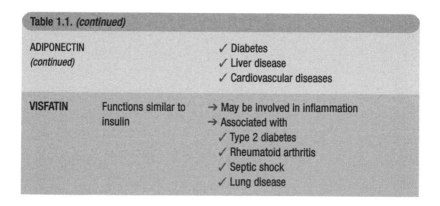

Table 1.1. *(continued)*		
ADIPONECTIN *(continued)*		✓ Diabetes ✓ Liver disease ✓ Cardiovascular diseases

VISFATIN	Functions similar to insulin	→ May be involved in inflammation
		→ Associated with
		  ✓ Type 2 diabetes
		  ✓ Rheumatoid arthritis
		  ✓ Septic shock
		  ✓ Lung disease

Because arthritis is an inflammatory process, increased levels of fat hormones can lead to both forms of arthritis. In addition to the inflammation caused by these fat-produced chemicals, osteoarthritis in dogs is also caused by the oxidative stress and activation of the flow of inflammatory compounds associated with obesity. We still have years of research ahead before the deepest and hardest questions about obesity and arthritis are answered. For now, dog owners should understand that crippling joint pain and irreversible damage are directly and indirectly caused by excess weight. While we're a long way from a cure for arthritis, there is hope. Today, we can focus on what we know works to reduce the risk of arthritis in dogs: avoiding extra pounds and losing them.

Increased Oxidative Stress

With age comes the opportunity for disease. Just because your dog gets older doesn't mean it will develop a serious medical condition; advanced age only increases the likelihood of illness. While many of us have come to accept illness, loss of physical function, weakness, and decline as inevitable attributes of age, very little scientific evidence proves that this *must* happen. Of course, living is a tough business for everyone; after all, the known mortality rate is 100 percent. Rather than focus exclusively on how long we or our dogs live in years, we should focus on living as long as possible in the most vibrant and active manner possible. The famous physician and originator of aerobics, Dr. Kenneth Cooper, calls this "squaring off the curve." Dr. Cooper describes life as a curve leading up to optimal health, reaching a plateau for decades, and then a sudden drop-off, culminating in a quick demise—squaring the curve instead of a long and gradual decline during the last decade or two of life. Born in 1931 and still an active runner, or "cooper" as it is known in Brazil after his techniques helped him lead Pelé and the Brazilian soccer team to the 1970 World Cup title, Dr. Cooper has logged a reported 38,000 miles and counting. My goal is not only to square off the lives of my pet patients, but to do the same in my own life as well as the lives of my family.

The ravages of time come from a multitude of factors, chief among them the cumulative effects of oxidative stress. Oxidative stress can result in damage to an organism's DNA, increasing the risk of disease and cancer. In effect, the longer an organism lives, the more cellular damage potentially accumulates until the cells reach a point of failure. This process could result in conditions such as diabetes, heart disease, and many forms of cancer.

Obesity increases the risk of oxidative damage. In fact, some research concludes that it is not the passage of time that causes damage but rather the accumulation of fat. In a 2003 study conducted by Boston University and the National Institutes of Health, scientists found that aging was not necessarily associated with higher oxidative stress and damage. Older, overweight, and obese individuals showed more evidence of oxidative stress than their leaner counterparts. What they found was that it isn't just getting older that leads to oxidative stress but the condition your body is in as you age. Leaner people had less oxidative damage, living longer with fewer diseases. Sounds good to me.

Some veterinary scientists and dog owners think that because dogs don't live as long, they may not experience as much oxidative stress. The 2003 study seems to contradict that notion. As our understanding of aging and disease increases, we may find that our dog's bodies are well-equipped to handle the damage of normal, everyday oxidation of living but not very good at combating the damaging effects of obesity-related oxidation.

In an April 2009 study published in the *Journal of Animal Physiology and Animal Nutrition*, researchers compared ten obese dogs with ten normal-weight dogs. The researchers, primarily from the University of Tennessee College of Veterinary Medicine, suggest that obesity in dogs is associated with increased oxidative stress, confirming earlier studies in children, rats, and other species. The obese dogs were found to have more DNA damage than normal-weight dogs. Further, researchers found that normal defense mechanisms against oxidative damage were diminished in obese dogs.

Obese dogs are in a state of perpetual low-grade inflammation as a result of the damaging chemicals that excess fat tissue secretes. This chronic inflammation leads to oxidative stress and plays a critical role in how many diseases develop. I often tell my clients, "If a person had a fever for several years and did nothing about it, you'd call them nuts. Further, you'd expect that same feverish person to have all sorts of serious medical problems." A fever is another way your body responds to inflammation. Most of the damage lies well beneath the outward sign of an increased body temperature. Obese dogs, and people for that matter, are living a life similar to an endless fever. Eventually the damage surfaces in the form of a nasty ailment. Sometimes the dog will become crippled, sometimes they will get cancer, and other times it's deadly high blood pressure; either way, these diseases always take our beloved friends before their time.

Diabetes

Obesity has long been linked with the development of diabetes mellitus in humans. Is there a link between obesity and diabetes in dogs? The answer is: sort of.

The two main types of diabetes are Type 1, also known as "diabetes mellitus type 1," "juvenile-onset diabetes," and "insulin-dependent diabetes"; and Type 2 diabetes mellitus, also called "adult-onset" or "non-insulin-dependent" diabetes. In Type 1 diabetes the body isn't making any insulin, while Type 2 diabetics are making insulin, just not enough. Type 1 occurs independently of weight while Type 2 is often caused by obesity.

Unfortunately, these terms are used to describe diabetes in humans and don't clearly translate for our common household pets. The type of diabetes seen in dogs is closer to Type 1 but has some characteristics of Type 2. Confused? You're not alone. A more accurate terminology would be "canine diabetes" and "feline diabetes."

Because we continue to use the human nomenclature, however, Type 1 diabetes is the most frequently seen form in dogs. It occurs when the body fails to produce adequate insulin to regulate blood sugar (glucose) levels. Type 1 diabetes is said to be insulin-dependent because it occurs when the pancreas fails to produce enough insulin. "Non-insulin-dependent" means that the pancreas is producing adequate insulin but something is interfering with its function. When we apply the human definition for Type 1 diabetes as having antibodies against the beta-cells of the pancreas that produce insulin, about half of diabetic dogs would be classified as Type 1 diabetics. The remainder of diabetic dogs would be classified as having other forms: (1) resulting from damage to the pancreas (about 28 percent), (2) diestrus-induced (similar to gestational or pregnancy-induced diabetes), and (3) chronic insulin-resistance. The last term, chronic insulin-resistance, interests us the most in the link between obesity and diabetes in dogs.

Contrary to what you may have heard, we don't have scientific evidence to link obesity with Type 2 diabetes in dogs, the form of diabetes most commonly seen in overweight humans. For some unknown reason, obese dogs don't tend to get Type 2 diabetes. Cats, however, do tend to get type 2 diabetes, similar to obese humans.

So the next time you hear someone say "Fat dogs get diabetes," you'll know that the statement may not be entirely true. In dogs, the link between excess weight and diabetes is not fully recognized, but the effect obesity has on canine insulin receptors is now being closely examined. It's all word-play, but until we re-define diabetes, we can only associate obesity with insulin resistance, not Type 2 diabetes.

Insulin Resistance

Obesity is known to cause insulin resistance in dogs. In simple terms, insulin works like this: a dog eats a meal, the body senses the increase in blood sugar, and the pancreas secretes insulin. Insulin is necessary to allow fat and muscle cells to absorb and store the sugar. As the sugar enters the fat and muscle cells, the decreasing blood glucose levels signal the pancreas to stop producing insulin.

In obese dogs, the number of insulin receptors on the fat and muscle cells are reduced, damaged, or don't function normally. There are several proposed reasons for this, and research is under way to discover the true cause. Regardless, because there are too few properly working insulin receptors, the body is fooled into thinking it doesn't have adequate insulin and therefore secretes more insulin, a condition called hyperinsulinemia. Even worse, because the abnormal receptors don't correctly bind insulin, the glucose is often left circulating, resulting in high blood sugar or hyperglycemia. While not the type of diabetes commonly seen in obese humans, insulin resistance in dogs often eventually leads to diabetes. The theory is that the insulin-secreting beta cells of the pancreas fail over time. We currently believe this is due to prolonged and high demand on the pancreas to produce insulin, oxidative damage, or the toxic effects of persistent high blood sugar on the beta cells. The result is that the pancreas becomes unable to produce enough insulin resulting in diabetes.

The take-home message is that the relationship between insulin, obesity, and longevity is intimately intertwined. A 2003 study published in the *Journal of Nutrition* concluded that the more efficient a dog is at removing glucose from the blood after a meal, the longer its life expectancy and the higher its quality of life. In other words, the more sensitive a dog is to insulin, as opposed to the obese dog's lack of response to insulin, the longer it lived. Dogs found to be more insulin sensitive were thinner and ate fewer calories. If you want your dog to avoid the rigors of insulin resistance and possible complications of diabetes, do it a favor and put it on a weight-loss program and feed it low-glycemic-index foods such as meat and fish, whole grains, and vegetables.

High Blood Pressure

Most dogs with high blood pressure or hypertension exhibit no clinical signs, which is why hypertension is referred to as the "silent killer." High blood pressure damages every organ system slowly and surely. The most common clinical sign of high blood pressure in humans is a headache. The most common clinical sign in dogs is, unfortunately, sudden blindness or loss of vision secondary to retinal damage. Dog owners who wait to take action until signs of high blood pressure develop are waiting until catastrophe strikes in the form of major organ damage or failure. You simply won't know your dog has high blood pressure until it's too late, unless your veterinarian checks for it.

The veterinary community still does not agree on what constitutes normal blood pressure for dogs. Blood pressure is reported in terms of *systolic* (when the heart is contracting or pumping blood—the first number), *diastolic* (when the heart is resting or not pumping blood—the second number), and *mean* arterial pressure (MAP) (the average of systolic and diastolic pressures). The accepted normal blood pressure range for dogs is a systolic pressure between 120 and 180 mm Hg (millimeters of mercury, the units used to measure blood pressure), mean blood pressure around 70 to 90 mm Hg, and diastolic pressure of 30 to 50 mm Hg. Another way to represent these values in dogs is 120–180/30–50 mm Hg with a MAP 70–90 mm Hg. The wide ranges are the result of our lack of big studies, variations in breeds, and nervousness of our pet patients. Many doctors, including myself, believe the normal blood pressure for dogs is closer to 120–140/70–80 mm Hg, very similar to humans. A dog with a systolic blood pressure of 160 mm Hg worries me from a hypertensive standpoint. If the patient is extremely nervous, we'll often repeat the reading on another day in another setting to determine if the hypertension is real or the result of anxiety and nervousness. It is not uncommon for dogs to have a falsely elevated blood pressure that returns to normal after a few minutes of calming down or during a different visit.

In the past decade, more small-animal veterinarians have begun monitoring blood pressure in dogs, leading to an increase in the reported cases of hypertension. For years, mainly because of the limitations of techniques and technology combined with our limited comprehension of blood pressure in dogs, it simply wasn't routinely checked in the general practice environment. That's changed now, and many dogs have their blood pressure monitored during anesthesia and surgery, as part of examinations for senior wellness, and for heart disease and obesity patients.

As the human obesity epidemic exploded into uncharted realms, the number of patients with high blood pressure also skyrocketed. Estimates are now that up to 30 percent of American adults have high blood pressure. Of those 30 percent with hypertension, 65 to 75 percent are directly related to excess weight. We're seeing the same problems in dogs.

A March 2003 *Hypertension* study looked at dogs fed a high-fat diet and the consequences weight gain had on blood pressure. Fifteen beagles were used in the nine-week study: six control-group dogs were fed a normal diet and maintained a lean body weight, and nine study dogs were fed a high-fat diet. The high-fat-diet group was fed as much maintenance diet mixed with uncooked beef fat as they wanted. And did they eat! The control group gained only about a half-pound during the nine-week study, while the high-fat group gained almost 3 pounds! These dogs aren't that different from our indoor pooches fed a normal diet and given treats and goodies from the table every day.

The experimental beagles were found to have a starting average systolic blood pressure of 143 to 145 mm Hg, diastolic pressure of 79 mm Hg, and mean arterial pressure of 100 mm Hg. After nine weeks, the normal-diet dogs had systolic blood pressure of 148 mm hg and diastolic pressure of 80 mm Hg. The control-study dogs' blood pressures changed very little during the study period.

Not so with the now-overweight dogs. Their blood pressure jumped to a systolic rate of 161 mm Hg and diastolic rate of 92 mm Hg. The mean arterial pressure in the dogs maintained on a normal diet and weight was 102 mm Hg, while the high-fat-diet dogs escalated to 115 mm Hg.

Table 13.1. Blood Pressure in Dogs

	Systolic Blood Pressure (mm Hg)	Diastolic Blood Pressure (mm Hg)	Mean Arterial Pressure (mm Hg)
Normal range for dogs	120 to 180	30 to 50	70 to 90
Mississippi study mixed-breed dogs at start of study	128	66	83
Mississippi study mixed-breed dogs high-fat, high-calorie diet and weight gain after five weeks	149	80	100
French study beagles— start of study	143 to 145	79	100 to 101
French study beagles normal diet and weight for nine weeks	148	80	102
French study beagles high-fat, high-caloric diet and weight gain for nine weeks	161	92	115

Finally, the hormone leptin may also play a role in obesity-related hypertension. Elevated blood levels of leptin have been associated with high blood pressure in rats. An article published in the June 2006 issue of *Vascular Health Risk Management* concluded that, while we don't fully understand how leptin causes hypertension, it does appear to be involved and may act on the kidneys, resulting in sodium retention and constriction of blood vessels.

We still have considerable basic science ahead of us to completely comprehend the relationship between obesity and high blood pressure. For now, the link has been clearly established in dogs: overweight dogs often develop high blood pressure. Dogs fed a high-fat, high-calorie diet gain weight and begin to develop damaging side effects in as little as two weeks. I expect that high blood pressure in overweight dogs will become a hot topic for veterinarians and dog owners over the next decade. If you're considering a weight-loss program for your dog, keep in mind that the dangerous consequences of even a few extra pounds begin quickly and worsen even quicker.

Heart Disease and High Cholesterol

As far back as the sixth century BC, Sushutra, the pioneer of Indian medicine, had made the connection between obesity and heart problems. In fact, when you think of obesity in people, the most likely complication you'll think of is heart disease. We are generally referring to the buildup of cholesterol plaques in the blood vessels, especially the blood vessels that supply the heart muscle. This condition is called atherosclerosis, and it affects about 5 million Americans. If the heart blood vessels become severely blocked, chest pain—angina—often develops, and if left untreated, a myocardial infarct or heart attack may result.

For our pet dogs, the situation is not exactly the same. When a dog has high blood fats (lipids) or cholesterol, it has been traditionally thought to be secondary to another illness, such as Cushing's disease, hypothyroidism, liver disease, or a nephropathy (kidney disease). There are two primary causes of high blood fats or lipid disorders (not caused by another disease or diet) in dogs: idiopathic hyperlipidemia (unknown cause of high blood fats) in miniature schnauzers and hypercholesterolemia in briards.

Obesity has only been recently indicated as a cause of high blood fats and cholesterol in dogs. The plain and simple reasons that high blood fats haven't been more vigorously investigated are that the dog isn't an ideal experimental model for human heart disease and dogs typically don't live long enough to encounter the blood-vessel blockages that years of high triglycerides and cholesterol create. Both of these assumptions have recently been reconsidered. Just because dogs may not have heart attacks as humans do, it doesn't follow that we should necessarily ignore their cholesterol levels.

Obese dogs and dogs fed high-fat diets have high cholesterol and triglyceride levels. A 2005 study conducted by the Animal Nutrition Unit of the Veterinary Faculty of the University of Liege in Belgium found that obese dogs fed as much as they wanted had higher levels of blood cholesterol and triglycerides—as much as 41 percent higher than lean dogs. In addition, their "bad cholesterol" or low-density lipoprotein (LDL) and very low-density lipoprotein (VLDL) were 58 percent and 125 percent higher, respectively. Their triglyceride levels were 75 percent higher than a normal-weight control dog.

After one month of being fed the high-protein, low-calorie diet, the obese dogs' total cholesterol dropped 16 percent, LDL plummeted 53 percent, VLDL decreased 44 percent, and triglycerides improved 48 percent.

The importance of these findings has many practical implications for your dog. If you feed a low-fat, low-calorie diet and keep your dog lean, cholesterol levels remain lower. While we don't yet know all the long-term health consequences of high blood fats in dogs, we suspect they cause similar damage to that seen in humans. We also know that high cholesterol has been associated with several eye problems, caused at least in part by the excess circulating blood fats depositing in the eye and tiny blood vessels of the eye.

We've also known since the 1970s that high triglyceride levels in dogs can cause acute pancreatitis, especially in obese dogs and in miniature schnauzers with a hereditary history of high blood fats. Atherosclerosis (thickening of the arteries from a buildup of fatty materials) is rare in dogs but has been seen in dogs with high cholesterol levels secondary to diabetes or that are being fed a high-fat diet. When a dog's cholesterol level is above 19 mmol/L or 700 mg/dl (less than 8 mmol/L or 300 mg/dl is normal), your dog is in the cholesterol danger zone.

Why don't dogs get atherosclerosis? Much of the mystery was solved in the 2005 Belgium study. The same obese dogs with high cholesterol, LDL, and VLDL levels also had remarkably high "good cholesterol" or high-density lipoprotein (HDL). For reasons we don't yet understand, the obese dogs had 45 percent higher HDL levels than their lean study partners. The protective ability of HDL is postulated as the reason that obese dogs don't get atherosclerosis the way humans do. Research is now examining why overweight dogs produce more protective HDL. Perhaps the solution to human heart disease may lie within our canine companions after all.

Obesity may also lead to damage of the heart itself. One of my chief concerns is that dogs, like people, are becoming obese at earlier and earlier ages. Because the damage associated with obesity is cumulative and progressive, the longer a dog is overweight, the more likely obesity-related diseases become. One of the primary ways muscle tissue, including heart muscle, becomes damaged is by oxidative stress. A November 2003 *Obesity Research* journal review discussed the multitude of relationships between obesity, insulin resistance, and heart disease. The author, Dr. Enrique Caballero of Harvard Medical School, sums it up as follows: "Obesity and insulin resistance damage the blood vessels and lead to diabetes and heart disease." Because overweight dogs are known to develop insulin resistance, these changes are also most likely occurring in obese dogs.

Respiratory Disease

Obesity can also cause respiratory problems in dogs. The presence of excess fat along the chest wall and abdomen compresses the spongy lungs, causing a reduction in the amount of air taken in with each breath. In many ways, this is similar to having a heavy bag pushing down on your chest; catching your breath becomes incredibly difficult. This excess fat also alters the normal breathing pattern, resulting in uneven and jerky breathing. Many obese dogs pant excessively after even a short walk in a desperate attempt to gain more oxygen. In more severe obesity, a ventilation-perfusion abnormality may occur, which is basically a dangerous situation in which not enough oxygen is entering into the body but the dog still has normal arterial carbon dioxide levels. This condition usually occurs with other problems, such as congenital heart defects. It's hard to imagine that obesity can cause the same respiratory distress as a major birth defect.

A June 2007 study published in the *Journal of the American Veterinary Medical Association* found that obese dogs experienced breathing problems when they exhaled. This was only evident when the dogs breathed rapidly. The dogs in this study were privately owned pet retrievers, the same type of dog with which you may share your home. The researchers also found that the respiratory problems increased as the dogs studied became more obese. Their findings indicate that the breathing problems of obese dogs may be more related to the lower airway (lungs) that the upper airway (throat and windpipe).

As obesity progresses, obese dogs may also experience a form of sleep apnea, similar to that of overweight humans.

Tracheal collapse is also frequently seen in overweight dogs, especially obese toy breeds. This may be due to primary compression of the fragile trachea by excess fat, weakened tracheal cartilage rings due to increased cortisol or damaging adipocytokines secreted by fat, increased inspiratory effort due to obesity, or a combination of all three. There is very little help for a dog with tracheal collapse other than weight reduction. Many owners of dogs with collapsing trachea fail to recognize the critical role that excess weight plays in the development or exacerbation of the condition. If your dog is diagnosed with collapsing trachea and the dog is even a pound overweight, help your dog shed excess weight.

Respiratory distress related to excess fat is different than brachycephalic airway syndrome. Obese dogs rarely snort, gurgle, or otherwise have noisy breathing. The vast majority of obese dogs are able to compensate for any decreased respiration while resting, making the image of the "fat, lazy, sleeping dog" an accurate one. Put that same dog on a leash and go for a run and you have a different picture: "fat, lazy, and collapsed dog."

Cruciate Ligament Injury

The cranial cruciate ligament is one of two fibrous bands of tissue that cross inside the knee joint, hence the name "cruciate," which means "cross." The function of the cranial and caudal cruciate ligaments is to stabilize the lower leg and help prevent it from moving in front of the upper leg when standing and moving. The cranial cruciate ligament is analogous to the anterior cruciate ligament in humans. This is one of the most common ligament injuries in dogs (and human athletes). The risk of cranial cruciate ligament rupture is higher in certain breeds of dogs, such as the Rottweiler, Labrador and Chesapeake Bay retrievers, Newfoundland, Akita, Neapolitan mastiff, Saint Bernard, and Staffordshire bull terrier. Some veterinary surgeons have postulated that this condition is due to changes in the angles of the bones of the knee joint. This suggestion has not been conclusively proven, and many dogs with very steep angles in their knees do not have as a high an incidence of cruciate injuries as others. Spaying and neutering has also been implicated to increase the risk for cruciate injury, more in females than males. The reason for this increase is unclear at this time and may be a matter of statistical aberration or that most dogs in the United States are spayed and neutered. Dogs weighing more than 50 pounds have been shown to be at greater risk of cruciate injury and tend to develop problems at an earlier age than smaller dogs.

Obesity is also suspected as a risk factor for cranial cruciate rupture, although scientific studies have not been clear on the role excess weight plays in these injuries. I suspect the same cartilage-damaging compounds and hormones associated with obesity in people also contribute to the weakening and alteration of the cruciate ligaments in dogs. Combined with the increased load and force of excess weight, it's no wonder that chronic cruciate ligament injuries are believed to be the most common cause of rear leg lameness in dogs. According to a 2005 report in the *Journal of the American Veterinary Medical Association*, Americans spent an estimated $1.32 billion on treatment for ruptured cranial cruciate ligaments in 2003. In a 2008 report from Veterinary Pet Insurance, over 1 million dogs were treated for cruciate ligament injuries, costing their owners over $1,500 each. If nothing else motivates you to help your dog lose weight, perhaps the economic cost of treating an overweight dog's knee injury will move you to take preventive action.

Kidney Disease

You've already learned that excess weight in dogs leads to high blood pressure. The organ that receives approximately one-quarter of the blood pumped out by the heart is the kidney. High blood pressure, therefore, directly and severely impacts this vital organ. Several studies as far back as 1989 have linked obesity with kidney disease. Research published in a 2005 edition of *Hypertension* proved that dogs experienced altered kidney function when they were fed a high-fat diet and allowed to gain weight. It took only five weeks of being fed dog food with added cooked beef fat to make the dogs obese and cause structural damage to their kidneys. More worrisome is the fact that this damage may not be completely reversible if the excess weight is lost. A 2004 German study found that some obese dogs that lost weight regained normal kidney function, while others still had signs of kidney disease, such as the presence of protein in the urine (microalbuminuria/proteinuria) and hypertension. These dogs required lifelong medical treatment.

Additional research is needed to determine the exact extent obesity plays in kidney disease and the improvement, if any, that weight loss has on obesity-related kidney disease.

Cancer

For the past twenty years, the relationship between obesity and certain cancers has been established. Cancers of the colon, breast (in postmenopausal women), endometrium (the inner lining of the uterus), kidney, and esophagus have all been linked to obesity in humans. Newer research has reported that obesity may cause cancers of the gallbladder, ovaries, and pancreas. Morbidly obese males have recently been reported as developing breast cancer due to the estrogen-like compounds secreted by fat. The National Cancer Institute estimates that obesity and physical inactivity may account for 25 to 30 percent of many major cancers.

The debate on the fat/cancer link is whether the fat cells promote cancer or that the obesity-related insulin resistance is to blame. A fascinating 2007 study published in *Cancer Research* found that high levels of insulin, insulin-like growth factor-1, and pro-inflammatory cytokines may be the true cause of the higher rates of cancer associated with obesity. The bottom line is that obesity in linked with increased cancer, at least in mice and men. We just don't understand exactly how.

Unfortunately we don't have cancer studies in dogs as we do for humans. Tumor development in dogs may be due to chronic infection or inflammation. We know obese dogs are in a constant state of low-grade inflammation and that fat secretes many dangerous compounds which may promote tumor development and growth. What we don't have are studies that follow obese dogs to see if they develop cancer more frequently than lean dogs. Veterinarians are beginning to report diagnosing breast cancer in obese spayed females. This was once unknown in spayed dogs. Veterinary oncologists include obesity on their lists of risk factors for cancer in dogs. I expect studies in the near future will parallel those conducted in humans that prove the link between excess fat tissue and cancer.

Overweight dogs are most likely at risk for developing many forms of cancer. Lose the weight; reduce the risk.

Skin Diseases

Obesity has long been associated with many skin problems in humans. Obesity causes changes in hormones or secretes substances that may cause *acanthosis nigricans*, which are darkened, velvety areas of the neck and body folds. Chronic stretching of the skin may result in stretch marks known as *striae*. Increased blood pressure in the leg veins may cause fluid retention and swelling of the legs; rupture of tiny, superficial vessels called capillaries leading to capillaritis; the development of varicose veins; inflammation of the skin or dermatitis; and even skin ulcers. Moisture that is trapped within rolls of fat or body folds creates an ideal environment for the growth of bacteria and fungi, leading to skin rashes and many types of infections, known as *intertrigo*. The good news is that many of these skin problems go away with weight loss.

In dogs, the connection between obesity and skin disease is just being determined. Veterinary dermatologists report that obesity is a risk factor for many skin conditions. A 2009 Japanese study evaluated 4,005 dogs and found that dogs with a body fat percentage greater than 35 had 2.4 times the incidence of fungal ear infections and 1.84 times the number of bacterial skin infections or pyoderma compared to dogs with less than 35 percent body fat.

Urinary Incontinence

Many women are familiar with the term "stress incontinence." If you're not, here it is in a nutshell: urine leaks out whenever you cough, sneeze, laugh out loud, or lift a heavy object. It's a real problem, not to mention embarrassing, for many women. In an August 2005 study, obesity was found to be significantly more common in women with stress incontinence than in the normal-weight population. This is thought to be due to increased pressure on the bladder from surrounding abdominal fat. Many surgeons now require women to lose weight prior to performing corrective surgery.

The same relationship between abdominal fat and urinary incontinence in dogs is suspected. While many cases of urinary incontinence in dogs are unrelated to obesity, a growing concern is that obesity may cause or worsen incontinence.

Reproductive Problems

The vast majority of pet dogs in the United States are spayed or neutered. For dogs used for breeding purposes, being overweight may lead to infertility and birthing problems (dystocia). Scientists have not understood why this occurs, but a 2009 Australian study published in the *Journal of Clinical Endocrinology & Metabolism* offers one reason. Researchers found that the inflammation caused by excess abdominal fat (white adipose tissue) may alter the ovarian environment leading to infertility despite apparently normal menstrual cycles. These same changes are likely to occur in obese dogs.

Decreased Wound Healing and Surgical Complications

A chief complaint among veterinary and human surgeons is that obese patients don't heal well. Whether the cause is increased tension along an incision site caused by excess fat or if the inflammatory chemicals produced by fat slow the healing process, the simple fact is that obese patients have more postoperative complications. A March 2007 study in the *World Journal of Surgery* demonstrated that obese human patients have a significantly higher risk of complications after surgery, including heart attack, wound infection, nerve injury, and urinary tract infection. The researchers also found that morbidly obese patients had a death rate almost twice as high as that of all other hospital patients.

Studies such as this are lacking in dogs, but anecdotal evidence abounds. Even without solid scientific evidence or clinical studies, many veterinarians are reluctant to perform a variety of surgical procedures on massively obese dogs for fear of unforeseeable and unavoidable complications.

Anesthetic Complications

As human surgeries involve more and more obese patients, the recognition of obesity-related anesthetic complications has arisen. A March 2008 *Clinician's Brief* warned veterinarians that obese dogs carried an increased anesthetic risk. As mentioned earlier in the book, I often tell the owners of healthy-weight dogs that their dog is "ER-ready": if their dog requires emergency surgery or treatment, their chances of survival are excellent. I only wish I could say the same for the other half of my patients—the overweight and obese dogs that are ER-ready only in the sense that they are headed to the emergency room sooner than later.

• • •

Duffy's Demise

Not all stories of overweight dogs have a happy ending. By the time Duffy made it to my office for a second opinion, she was in bad shape. Years of carrying around too much weight had taken their toll. She was near the end and could barely manage to wag her tail. Her pet parent had heard about our clinic's success with older obese pets and was hoping for a miracle. As I began Duffy's exam, I hardly felt like a miracle worker.

Duffy was a petite mixed-breed dog. Somewhere along the line she picked up the genes of a dachshund, Yorkshire terrier, and a bit of beagle for good measure. If Duffy had been raised with a different diet and lifestyle, she would have weighed about 15 pounds. Instead she tipped our scales at 28 pounds. She was the equivalent of two dogs in one body, and the damage was apparent as I listened to her tiny heart struggle against the fat in her chest cavity.

Every movement was a struggle for Duffy. She could no longer hop onto the bed at night; her owner had to pick her up. Her blood sugar swung wildly despite high, twice-daily injections of insulin. Three times in the past six months she had gone into diabetic shock and almost died. Duffy's owner was looking for relief for her best friend.

Duffy's list of ailments was long— all of them caused and exacerbated by her weight: cataracts, periodontal disease, osteoarthritis, enlarged liver, dry flaky skin, diabetes, heart disease, respiratory distress, and diminished mental responsiveness. A challenging case would be a patient with any three of these maladies at one time. Duffy had them all and needed immediate help.

I knew Duffy's owner loved her deeply. If she didn't, she wouldn't have been in my office. Unfortunately, love isn't always enough. In fact, most of Duffy's problems were the result of being loved too much. Duffy's owner believed that the best way to demonstrate care and compassion was through food . . . cookies, treats, and table foods. She rationalized her actions by saying that Duffy gave so much and asked so little that surely she deserved a few "yum-yum's." What's the point in having a dog, she questioned, if you can't spoil it a little?

As I continued discussing Duffy's medical conditions, I could see the tears beginning to swell in the owner's eyes. She was doing her best to put on a brave face, trying to act as if she expected better news or that

I would offer a newly developed or experimental treatment, but I could sense she was beginning to accept there would be no help for Duffy.

Or was there?

Duffy was only five years old. Any other small mixed-breed dog would be in the prime of life. Duffy had all the diseases that we typically associate with very old patients. If you'd given me her medical record without any of Duffy's biographical information, I would've guessed she was fifteen or seventeen years old. Obesity caused or worsened every medical condition she had. All were preventable. Now every single one of them was making Duffy's life miserable. After almost four years of struggling day in and day out, Duffy and her human family were ready to give up.

All of the physical exam findings, scientific data, and medical history told me that Duffy was looking at six living another to twelve months, tops. My heart was breaking.

Not wanting to give up hope, I outlined an initial diet, exercise, and supplement plan, and changed her heart and pain management medications. We'd take it slow at first and then get more aggressive as Duffy's health and fitness improved. With additional diagnostic testing and a follow-up scheduled for the next week, I thought I saw a glimmer of hope in the owner's eyes.

Surprisingly, Duffy failed to show up for her examination the following week. My telephone message was unanswered. After two weeks and several unreturned calls to Duffy's owner, we received a nondescript letter.

Dear Dr. Ward, thank you for your interest and concern in Duffy. We decided not to pursue any further treatment for her after meeting with you. We took Duffy to our regular veterinarian and had her put to sleep. Thank you again.

A shiver spread through my entire body, and I grew faint. As I stared at the note, I felt as though someone had reached into my soul and torn out a chunk. I was no newcomer to losing patients, but this time it hurt deeply. For some reason Duffy had affected me even though I met her only once. Why had I failed? What should I have done differently? While some might say I was being too sensitive, that I needed to keep some space between myself and my patients, to me, this case wasn't just about Duffy but rather speaking the truth about preventive health care for pets. As a doctor, I was devastated. I had an obligation to speak up for my patients that can't speak for themselves. I follow a code of ethics that values truth above all else, including hurt feelings, regardless of whether they're mine or my client's. The truth is that Duffy's illnesses could've been prevented—without costly or painful surgery, but just by changing her diet and adding exercise.

I think about Duffy almost every time I'm dealing with an overweight or obese patient. I wonder if each of these clients will be sending me a note in the upcoming weeks or if I will find success. If my efforts result in one less "Duffy," then all the hard work and sacrifice will have been worthwhile.

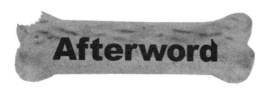

Afterword

OUR DOGS GIVE US SO MUCH. Unfortunately, too often we repay them for their unconditional love with too many treats and unhealthy foods that are causing them health problems. The purpose of this book is to inform, inspire, and enlighten dog owners to better care for your pet. After completing this book, you can help your dog and pets everywhere in these five ways.

1 Write your local political representatives and demand pet food manufacturers place calorie contents on their food in easy to read, as-fed amounts. At the very least we should be able to know how many calories are in a cup or a can. If enough concerned pet owners demand this simple change, the ramifications will extend far beyond the label.

Find your Representative:
https://writerep.house.gov
Contact your Senator:
http://www.senate.gov/general/contact_information/senators_cfm.cfm

2 Write to AAFCO and the FDA asking for better pet food labels and nutritional guidelines. As long as "natural" and "organic" mean whatever the pet food producer decides, pets pay the price. AAFCO needs to hear from pet owners, not just pet food companies.

AAFCO Board of Directors:
http://www.aafco.org/BoardofDirectors/tabid/61/Default.aspx

FDA Center for Veterinary Medicine:
240-276-9300
CVMHomeP@cvm.fda.gov
7519 Standish Place
HFV-12
Rockville, MD 20855

3 Walk your dog—daily. Perhaps nothing is as simple and benefi-cial as taking a walk. If each of the over 50 million dog owners walked their dog for 20 to 30 minutes each day, our nation's human and veterinary healthcare costs would be dramatically reduced. Commit to walking your dog—and yourself—daily.

4 Feed a healthy diet. Nourish your dog as you should nourish yourself.

5 Keep "The Promise." Cherish the time you have with your pet. Our dogs are with us for too brief a time; make the most of every day. Celebrate the unique relationship we've shared for tens of thousands of years. Your dog will live a longer and healthier life if you take better care of him or her. The most important thing you can do is to keep your dog at a healthy weight.

We're fortunate to share our lives with animals as complementary, interesting, and empathetic as dogs. In my opinion, this relationship is built into our DNA. Together we can make the world better a better place for future generations of people and pets.

Wags and purrs,
Dr. Ernie

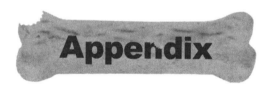

AAFCO Dog Food Nutrient Profiles

Below is a listing of the 2009 AAFCO Dog Food Nutrient Profiles. Any AAFCO-approved dog food must have a guaranteed analysis that meets or exceeds these values.

Nutrient	Units (dry-matter basis)	Growth and reproduction minimum	Adult maintenance minimum	Maximum
2009 AAFCO Dog Food Nutrient Profiles **Based on Dry Matter** *Presumes an energy density of 3500 kcal Metabolizable Energy/kilogram*				
CRUDE PROTEIN	%	22.0	18.0	
Arginine	%	0.62	0.51	
Histidine	%	0.22	0.18	
Isoleucine	%	0.45	0.37	
Leucine	%	0.72	0.59	
Lysine	%	0.77	0.63	
Methionine-cystine	%	0.53	0.43	
Phenylalanine-tyrosine	%	0.89	0.73	
Threonine	%	0.58	0.48	
Tryptophan	%	0.20	0.16	

Valine	%	0.48	0.39	
CRUDE FAT	%	8.0	5.0	
Linoleic acid	%	1.0	1.0	
MINERALS				
Calcium	%	1.0	0.6	2.5
Phosphorus	%	0.8	0.5	1.6
Ca:P ratio		1:1	1:1	2:1
Potassium	%	0.6	0.6	
Sodium	%	0.3	0.06	
Chloride	%	0.45	0.09	
Magnesium	%	0.04	0.04	0.3
IRON	mg/kg	80	80	3000
Copper	mg/kg	7.3	7.3	250
Manganese	mg/kg	5.0	5.0	
Zinc	mg/kg	120	120	1000
Iodine	mg/kg	1.5	1.5	50
Selenium	mg/kg	0.11	0.11	2
VITAMINS AND OTHER				
Vitamin A	IU/kg	5000	5000	250,000
Vitamin D	IU/kg	500	500	5000
Vitamin E	IU/kg	50	50	1000
Thiamine	mg/kg	1.0	1.0	
Riboflavin	mg/kg	2.2	2.2	
Pantothenic acid	mg/kg	10	10	
Niacin	mg/kg	11.4	11.4	
Pyridoxine	mg/kg	1.0	1.0	
Folic acid	mg/kg	0.18	0.18	
Vitamin B_{12}	mg/kg	0.022	0.022	
Choline	mg/kg	1200	1200	

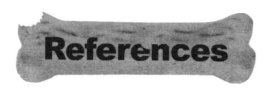

References

CHAPTER 1 Pet Obesity: A Supersized Problem

Lund, EM, Armstrong, PJ, Kirk, CA, and Klausner, JS. "Prevalence and Risk Factors for Obesity in Adult Dogs from Private US Veterinary Practices." *The International Journal of Applied Research in Veterinary Medicine.* 2006 Vol. 4, No. 2;177–186

Freeman, Lisa M, et al. "Disease prevalence among dogs and cats in the United States and Australia and proportions of dogs and cats that receive therapeutic diets or dietary supplements." *Journal of the American Veterinary Medical Association.* Aug 2006 15;229(4):531–4.

Lund, EM, Armstrong, PJ, Kirk, CA, and Klausner, JS. "Health status and population characteristics of dogs and cats examined at private veterinary practices in the United States." *Journal of the American Veterinary Medical Association.* May 1999 1;214(9):1336–41

Wohl, JS and Nusbaum, KE. "Public health roles for small animal practitioners." *Journal of the American Veterinary Medical Association.* Feb 2007 15;230(4):494–500

Association of Pet Obesity Prevention. "New Data Suggests that Pet Obesity is on the Rise." Calabash, NC. July 10, 2008. http://www.petobesityprevention.com/images/APOP%20Press%20Release %20July%20'08.pdf

Association of Pet Obesity Prevention. "Pet Obesity Expands In Us: Nationwide study finds half of dogs and cats now overweight or obese, an increase from 2007." Calabash, NC. February 10, 2009. http://www.petobesityprevention.com/images/APOP_Press_Release_Feb_2009.pdf

Naaz, Afia et al. "Loss of cyclin-dependent kinase inhibitors produces adipocyte hyperplasia and obesity." *The FASEB Journal.* 2004;18:1925–1927.

GS Hotamisligil, NS Shargill, and BM Spiegelman. "Adipose expression of tumor necrosis factor-alpha: direct role in obesity-linked insulin resistance." *Science* 1 January 1993 259: 87–91.

Herron, Daniel M. "C-reactive protein and adiposity: Obesity as a systemic inflammatory state." *Surgery for Obesity and Related Diseases.* Volume 1, Issue 3, May-June 2005, Pages 385–386.

Cottam, DR et al. "The chronic inflammatory hypothesis for the morbidity associated with morbid obesity: implications and effects of weight loss." *Obesity Surgery Journal.* 2004 May;14(5): 589–600.

Olefsky, Jerrold M. "IKKe: A Bridge between Obesity and Inflammation." *Cell.* Volume 138, Issue 5, 4 September 2009, Pages 834–836.

Trock, David. "Tired, Achy, and Overweight, the Inflammatory Nature of Obesity." *Journal of Clinical Rheumatology.* January 2009—Volume 15—Issue 1;50.

Miklósi, Ádám. "Dog Behavior, Evolution, and Cognition." Oxford, UK: Oxford University Press, 2007. Chapter 5, pages 95–136.

The Nielsen Company. "A2/M2 Three Screen Report: 1st Quarter 2009." http://blog.nielsen. com/nielsenwire/wp-content/uploads/2009/05/nielsen_threescreenreport_q109.pdf

Duty, Kim. "Apartment Living: The New American Dream?" National Multi Housing Council presentation. July 2002. http://www.nmhc.org/Content/ServeContent.cfm?IssueID=10&Content ItemID=1828&siteArea=Topics

CHAPTER 2 Marketing Addiction: The Epidemic of Kibble Crack

Case, Linda. "The Dog: Its Behavior, Nutrition, and Health." Ames, Iowa.: Blackwell Publishing Professional, 2005. Page 58.

Bureau of Labor Statistics American Time Use Survey and ERS Eating and Health Module. Updated date: June 15, 2009. http://www.ers.usda.gov/data/atus/

Levesque, A. "The sense of taste in dogs and cats." *Point Veterinaire.* Oct-Nov. 1997. Vol. 28(186); 45–53

Levin, Barry E., Ambrose A. Dunn-Meynell, Bork Balkan, and Richard E. Keesey. "Selective breeding for diet-induced obesity and resistance in sprague-dawley rats." *American Journal of Physiology—Regulatory, Integrative and Comparative Physiology.* Vol 273, Issue 2 725–R730

Colantuoni, C. et al. "Evidence That Intermittent, Excessive Sugar Intake Causes Endogenous Opioid Dependence." *Obesity Research.* Vol. 10 No. 6 June 2002:478–88

Sage JR, Knowlton BJ. "Effects of US devaluation on win-stay and win-shift radial maze performance in rats." *Behavioral Neuroscience.* 2000 Apr;114(2):295–306.

Volkow, ND and Wise, RA. "How can drug addiction help us understand obesity?" *Nature Neuroscience* 8, 555—560 (2005)

Thanos, PK et al. "Differences in response to food stimuli in a rat model of obesity: in-vivo assessment of brain glucose metabolism." *International Journal of Obesity.* 2008 Jul;32(7):1171–1179.

Lane, CH. "Dog Shows and Doggy People." London, UK.: Hutchinson and Company, 1902. Pages 224–225

Skinner, B. F. *The Behavior of Organisms: An Experimental Analysis.* Cambridge, Massachusetts: B. F. Skinner Foundation. 1938.

Kumazawa, T and Kurihara, K. "Large enhancement of canine taste responses to sugars by salts." *The Journal of General Physiology.* Vol. 95, 1007–1018.

Wise, Roy A. "Role of brain dopamine in food reward and reinforcement." *Philosophical Transactions of the Royal Society: Biological Science.* July 29, 2006 vol. 361 no. 1471 1149–1158.

Kuo, ZY. "The Dynamics of Behaviour Development: An Epigentic View." New York, NY.: Random House, 1967

Bradshaw, J and Thorne, C. "The Waltham Book of Dog and Cat Behavior." New York, NY.: Pergamon Press,1992. Feeding Behavior pages 115–129.

Mistretta, Charlotte M. et al. "Development of Gustatory Organs and Innervating Sensory Ganglia." *Chemical Senses.* 2005 Vol. 30(Supplement 1):i52–i53

Smotherman WP. "In utero chemosensory experience alters taste preferences and corticosterone responsiveness." *Behavioral and Neural Biology.* Vol. 36: 61–68, 1982

Euromonitor International. "Pet Food and Pet Care Products in the US." http://www.euromonitor. com/Pet_Food_And_Pet_Care_Products_in_the_US

American Pet Products Association (APPA). "Industry Statistics & Trends." http://www.american petproducts.org/press_industrytrends.asp

Mintel. "Pet Food and Supplies—US—July 2009."

Taylor, Jessica. "Riding Out the Recession." PetFoodIndustry.com. Sept. 30, 2009. http://www.pet foodindustry.com/ViewArticle.aspx?id=25980&terms=dog+food+sales

Mowat FM, et al. "Topographical characterization of cone photoreceptors and the area centralis of the canine retina. *Molecular Vision.* 2008; 14:2518-27.

Torres, CL, Hickenbottom, SJ and Rogers, Q. "Palatability affects the percentage of metabolizable energy as protein selected by adult beagles." *The Journal of Nutrition.* Vol. 133:3516–3522.

Romsos, DR and Ferguson, D. "Regulation of protein intake in adult dogs." *Journal of the American Veterinary Medical Association.* Vol. 182:41–43

Torres, CL et al. "Palatability affects the percentage of metabolizable energy as protein selected by adult beagles." *The Journal of Nutrition.* Vol. 133:3516–3522

Houpt, Katherine, Hintz, Harold F. and Shepherd, Paul. "The role of olfaction in canine food preferences." *Chemical Senses.* Vol. 3: 281–290.

Colantuoni C, Schwenker J, McCarthy J, Rada P, Ladenheim B, Cadet JL, Schwartz GJ, Moran TH, Hoebel BG. "Excessive sugar intake alters binding to dopamine and mu-opioid receptors in the brain." *Neuroreport.* Nov 2001 Vol. 16;12(16):3549–52.

CHAPTER 3 What Is Your Dog Eating? Deciphering Pet Food Labels

DeHaven, WR. "Re: Docket No. 2007-N-0442—Opportunity for Public Input on Standards for Pet Food and Other Animal Feeds; Notice of Meeting." June 13, 2008 letter. American Veterinary Medicalk Association. Schaumburg, IL. http://www.avma.org/advocacy/federal/regulatory/food_safety/feed_standards_comments.pdf

2009 Official Publication of American Feed Control Officials Incorporated. 2009. ISBN 1-878341-21-9

AAFCO Pet Food and Specialty Pet Food Labeling Guide. Revised February 2008. ISBN 1-878341-16-2

Nestle, Marion. "Pet Food Politics: The Chihuahua in the coal mine." Berkeley and Los Angeles, CA.: University of California Press, 2008. Chapter 2 pages 15–26

Corbett, Senator Ellen M. Senate Judiciary Committee. Senate Bill 1773. April 14, 2008. http://info.sen.ca gov/pub/07-08/bill/sen/sb_1751-1800/sb_1773_cfa_20080416_132343_sen_comm.html

Organic Trade Association. "U.S. organic sales grow by a whopping 17.1 percent in 2008." May 4, 2009. http://www.organicnewsroom.com/2009/05/us_organic_sales_grow_by_a_who.html

Murray, Sean M., Patil, Avinash R., Fahey Jr., George C., Merchen, Neal R., and Hughes, Denzil M. "Raw and Rendered Animal By-Products as Ingredients in Dog Diets." *The Journal of Nutrition.* Vol. 128 No. 12 December 1998, pp. 2812S–2815S

Dzanis, David A. "Safety of Ethoxyquin in Dog Foods." *The Journal of Nutrition.* 1991 121: S163–S164

Bednar, GE et al. "Starch and Fiber Fractions in Selected Food and Feed Ingredients Affect Their Small Intestinal Digestibility and Fermentability and Their Large Bowel Fermentability In Vitro in a Canine Model." *Journal of Nutrition.* 2001;131:276–286

Twomey, LN et al. "The Use of Sorghum and Corn as Alternatives to Rice in Dog Foods." *The Journal of Nutrition.* 2002;132:1704S–1705S

Moore, ML, Fottler, HJ, Fahey, Jr., GC and Corbin, JE. "Utilization of Corn-Soybean Meal-Substituted Diets by Dogs." *Journal of Animal Science.* 1980 Vol. 50:892–896.

Gajda, M et al. "Corn hybrid affects in vitro and in vivo measures of nutrient digestibility in dogs." *Journal of Animal Science.* 2005. Vol. 83:160–171

Carciofi, AC et al. "Effects of six carbohydrate sources on dog diet digestibility and post-prandial glucose and insulin response." *Journal of Animal Physiology and Animal Nutrition.* Volume 92, Number 3, June 2008, pp. 326–336

Zicker, Steven C. "Evaluating Pet Foods: How confident are you when you recommend a commercial pet food?" *Topics in Companion Animal Medicine.* August 2008. Vol. 23, Issue 3; 121–126

Dzanis, David A. "Understanding Regulations Affecting Pet Foods." Topics in Companion Animal Medicine. August 2008. Vol. 23, Issue 3;117–120

CHAPTER 4 Rx 1: Assess Your Dog's Weight

Burkholder, William J. "Use of body condition scores in clinical assessment of the provision of optimal nutrition." *Journal of the American Veterinary Medical Association.* Sep 2000 1;217(5):650–4.

Mawby, Dianne I. "Comparison of Various Methods for Estimating Body Fat in Dogs." *Journal of the American Animal Hospital Association.* 200440:109–114.

German, Alexander J. "The Growing Problem of Obesity in Dogs and Cats." *The Journal of Nutrition.* July 2006 Vol. 136:1940S–1946S.

Weight ranges for breeds based on a variety of publications and breed standards by the American Kennel Club (AKC).

CHAPTER 5 Rx 2: Rule Out a Medical Problem

Scott-Moncrieff, J. Catharine, Glickman, Nita W., Glickman, Lawrence T. and HogenEsch, Harm "Lack of Association between Repeated Vaccination and Thyroiditis in Laboratory Beagles." *Journal of Veterinary Internal Medicine* Volume 20 Issue 4, Pages 818 – 821.

German, Alexander J. "The Growing Problem of Obesity in Dogs and Cats." *The Journal of Nutrition.* July 2006. Vol. 136:1940S–1946S,

Bruin,CDe, Meij, BP, et al. "Cushing's disease in dogs and humans." *Hormone Research.* January 2009;71 Suppl 1(0):140–3.

Dallman, Mary F., et al. "Chronic stress and obesity: A new view of 'comfort food'". *Proceedings of the National Academy of Sciences.* Sept 30, 2003 vol. 100 no. 20;11696–11701

Kuo,Lydia E, et al. "Neuropeptide Y acts directly in the periphery on fat tissue and mediates stress-induced obesity and metabolic syndrome." *Nature Medicine.* July 2007. Vol. 13 No. 7;803–11.

Impellizeri, JA, Tetrick, MA, Muir, P. "Effect of weight reduction on clinical signs of lameness in dogs with hip osteoarthritis." *Journal of the American Veterinary Medical Association.* Apr 2000 1;216 (7):1089–91.

Smith, GK, Paster, ER, Powers, MY, et al. "Lifelong diet restriction and radiographic evidence of osteoarthritis of the hip joint in dogs." *Journal of the American Veterinary Medical Association.* Sep 2006 1;229(5):690–3.

Bach, JF, et al. "Association of expiratory airway dysfunction with marked obesity in healthy adult dogs." *American Journal of Veterinary Research.* Jun 2007. Vol. 68(6);670–5.

Slupe,JL, Freeman, LM, and Rush, JE. "Association of body weight and body condition with survival in dogs with heart failure." *Journal of Veterinary Internal Medicine.* May-Jun 2008;22(3):561–5.

Bergman, Richard N et al. "Abdominal obesity: role in the pathophysiology of metabolic disease and cardiovascular risk." *American Journal of Medicine.* February 2007;120(2 Suppl 1):S3-8;S29-32.

Philip-Couderc, P et al. "Cardiac transcriptome analysis in obesity-related hypertension." *Hypertension.* Mar 2003;41(3):414–21.

Dhurandhar, NV et al. "Increased adiposity in animals due to a human virus." *International Journal of Obesity.* 2000. Vol 24; 989–996

Atkinson, Richard L. "Viruses as an Etiology of Obesity." *Mayo Clinic Proceedings.* October 2007 vol. 82 no. 10;1192–1198.

Lyons, MJ, Nagashima, K and Zabriskie, JB. "Animal models of postinfectious obesity: Hypothesis and review." *Journal of NeuroVirology.* 2002 Vol. 8; 1–5.

Fredriksson R, Hägglund M, Olszewski PK, Stephansson O, Jacobsson JA, Olszewska AM, Levine AS, Lindblom J, Schiöth HB. "The obesity gene, FTO, is of ancient origin, up-regulated during food deprivation and expressed in neurons of feeding-related nuclei of the brain." *Endocrinology.* May 2008;149(5):2062–71.

Yamka RM, KG Friesen, X Gao, S Malladi, S Al-Murrani, L Bernal. "The effects of weight loss on gene expression in dogs." *Journal of Veterinary Internal Medicine.* 2008;22:7412008 ACVIM Meeting, San Antonio.

Bāckhed, Fredrik et al. "The gut microbiota as an environmental factor that regulates fat storage." *Proceedings of the National Academy of Sciences of the United States of America*. November 2, 2004 Vol. 101. No. 44 15718–15723.

Sharma AM, Pischon T, Hardt S, Kunz I, Luft FC. "Hypothesis: Beta-adrenergic receptor blockers and weight gain: A systematic analysis." *Hypertension*. Feb 2001. Vol. 37(2);250–4.

Kulkarni SK, Kaur G. "Pharmacodynamics of drug-induced weight gain." *Drugs Today*. Aug 2001. Vol. 37(8);559–572.

Allison DB, Mentore JL, Heo M, et al. "Antipsychotic-induced weight gain: a comprehensive research synthesis." *American Journal of Psychiatry*. Nov 1999. Vol. 156;1686–1696.

Fava M. "Weight gain and antidepressants." *Journal of Clinical Psychiatry*. 2006:61 Supplement 11:37–41.

CHAPTER 6 Rx 3: Calculate Calories and Set Your Weight-Loss Goals

National Research Council. "Nutrient Requirements of Dogs and Cats." Washington, DC.; The National Academies Press, 2006. Chapter 3, pages 33–37.

Zentek, J. "Studies on the effect of feeding on the microbial metabolism in the intestinal tract of dogs." Habilitation thesis, Tieraerztliche Hochschule, Hanover. 1993.

National Research Council. "Nutrient Requirements of Dogs and Cats." Washington, DC.; The National Academies Press, 2006. Chapter 3, page 36.

Patil, AR, Bisby, TM. "Comparison of maintenance energy requirement of client-owned dogs and kennel dogs." Purina Nutrition Forum Proceedings, 2001.

Kienzle, Ellen. "Further Developments in the Prediction of Metabolizable Energy (ME) in Pet Food." *The Journal of Nutrition*. 2002. Vol. 132: 1796S–1798S.

Burger, Ivan "Energy Needs of Companion Animals: Matching Food Intakes to Requirements Throughout the Life Cycle." *The Journal of Nutrition*. 1994. Vol. 124: 2584S–2593S.

Burger, Ivan H. and Johnson, Janel V. "Dogs Large and Small: The Allometry of Energy Requirements within a Single Species." *The Journal of Nutrition*. 1991. Vol. 121: S18–S21.

Ahlstrøm, Øystein, et al. "Energy Expenditure and Water Turnover in Hunting Dogs: A Pilot Study." *The Journal of Nutrition*. 2006. Vol. 136: 2063S–2065S.

Hill, Richard C. "Challenges in Measuring Energy Expenditure in Companion Animals: A Clinician's Perspective." *The Journal of Nutrition*. 2006. Vol. 136: 1967S–1972S.

Harper, EJ. "Changing Perspectives on Aging and Energy Requirements: Aging, Body Weight and Body Composition in Humans, Dogs and Cats." *The Journal of Nutrition*. 1998. Vol. 128;2627S–2631S.

Roudebush P, Schoenherr, WD, Delaney, SJ. "An evidence-based review of the use of therapeutic foods, owner education, exercise, and drugs for the management of obese and overweight pets". *Journal of the American Veterinary Medical Association*. Sep 2008 1;233(5):717–25.

Yaissle, JE, Holloway, Buffington, T. "Evaluation of owner education as a component of obesity treatment programs for dogs." *Journal of the American Veterinary Medical Association*. June 15, 2004, Vol. 224, No. 12;1932–1935

CHAPTER 7 Rx 4: Choose the Right Commercial Diet

Witschi, Hanspeter R., Doherty, David G. "Butylated Hydroxyanisole and Lung Tumor Development in A/J Mice." *Toxicological Sciences*. Vol. 4 No. 5 pp. 795–801.

Ito N, Fukushima S, and Tsuda H. "Carcinogenicity and Modification of the Carcinogenic Response by bha, Bht, and Other Antioxidants." *Critical Reviews in Toxicology*. 1985, Vol. 15, No. 2, Pages 109–150.

Robertson, John L, Goldschmidt, Michael, et al., "Long-term renal responses to high dietary protein in dogs with 75% nephrectomy." *Kidney International* 1986 Vol. 29, 511–519.

Rehman, Zia-ur, and Shah, WH. "Thermal heat processing effects on antinutrients, protein and starch digestibility of food legumes." *Food Chemistry.* June 2005. Vol. 91, Issue 2;327–33.

Wrangham, Richard, and Conklin-Brittain, NancyLou. "Cooking as a biological trait." *Comparative Biochemistry and Physiology—Part A: Molecular & Integrative Physiology.* September 2003. Vol. 136, Issue 1;35–46.

U.S. Food and Drug Administration. "FDA Suspends Temporary Emergency Permit of Pet Food Maker." June 12, 2009. http://www.fda.gov/AnimalVeterinary/NewsEvents/CVMUpdates/ucm 166265.htm

Joffe, Daniel J. Schlesinger, Daniel P. "Preliminary assessment of the risk of Salmonella infection in dogs fed raw chicken diets." *Canadian Veterinary Journal.* 2002 June; 43(6): 441–442.

Strohmeyer, RA et al. "Evaluation of bacterial and protozoal contamination of commercially available raw meat diets for dogs." *Journal of the American Veterinary Medical Association* February 15, 2006, Vol. 228, No. 4, Pages 537–542.

Canadian Veterinary Medical Association. "Raw Food Diets for Pets—Canadian Veterinary Medical Association and Public Health Agency of Canada Joint Position Statement." November 2006. http://canadianveterinarians.net/ShowText.aspx?ResourceID=554

Public Health Agency of Canada Advisory. "Salmonella infection in humans linked to natural pet treats, raw food diets for pets." July 2005. http://www.phac-aspc.gc.ca/media/advisories_avis/salmonella-eng.php

U.S. Food and Drug Administration. "Safe Handling Tips for Pet Foods and Treats." February 20, 2009. http://www.fda.gov/ForConsumers/ConsumerUpdates/ucm048182.htm

U.S. Food and Drug Administration. "FDA Tips for Preventing Foodborne Illness Associated with Pet Food and Pet Treats." July 27, 2007. http://www.fda.gov/AnimalVeterinary/NewsEvents/CVMUpdates/ucm048030.htm

CHAPTER 8   Rx 5: Make Home Cooking Healthy

National Animal Poison Control Center. www.aspca.org/apcc.

Bravata, Dena M. et al. "Efficacy and Safety of Low-Carbohydrate Diets." *Journal of the American Medical Association.* April 9, 2003, Vol. 289 No. 14, pp. 1837–1850.

Bierer, Tiffany Linn, Bui, Linh M. "High-Protein Low-Carbohydrate Diets Enhance Weight Loss in Dogs." *The Journal of Nutrition.* 134:2087S–2089S.

German, Alexander J. et al. "A high protein high fibre diet improves weight loss in obese dogs." *The Veterinary Journal.* January 12, 2009.

Bierer, TL and Bu, LM. "High-Protein Low-Carbohydrate Diets Enhance Weight Loss in Dogs." *The Journal of Nutrition.* August 2004 Vol. 134:2087S–2089S

Blanchard, G. "Rapid Weight Loss with a High-Protein Low-Energy Diet Allows the Recovery of Ideal Body Composition and Insulin Sensitivity in Obese Dogs." *The Journal of Nutrition.* August 2004 Vol. 134:2148S–2150S

Wakshlag JJ, Barr SC, Ordway GA, Kallfelz FA, Flaherty CE, Christensen BW, et al. Effect of dietary protein on lean body wasting in dogs: correlation between loss of lean mass and markers of proteasome-dependent proteolysis. *Journal of Animal Physiology and Animal Nutrition.* Dec 2003. Vol. 87(11–12):408–20.

Helman, EE, Huff-Lonergan, E, Davenport, GM and Lonergan, SM. "Effect of dietary protein on calpastatin in canine skeletal muscle." *Journal of Animal Science.* 2003. Vol. 81:2199–2205.

Diez, M. et al. "Weight Loss in Obese Dogs: Evaluation of a High-Protein, Low-Carbohydrate Diet." *The Journal of Nutrition.* 2002 Vol. 132: 1685S–1687S

Hand, Thatcher, Remillard and Roudebush. "Small Animal Clinical Nutrition, 4th Edition." Marceline, MO. Walsworth Publishing Company, 2000. Chapter 3, pages 125–126.

Thompson, Angele. "Ingredients: Where Pet Food Starts." *Topics in Companion Animal Medicine*. August 2008. Vol. 23, Issue 3;127–132

CHAPTER 9 Rx 6: Get Fido Fit

Hite, HM, Hanson, NR, Conti, PA and Mattis, PA. "Effect of cage size on patterns of activity and health of Beagle dogs." *Laboratory Animal Science*. Vol 27:60–64.

Delude, LA. "Activity patterns and behavior of sled dogs." *Applied Animal Behavioral Science*. Vol. 15:161–168.

Berman, M, Dunbar, I. "The social behavior of free-ranging suburban dogs." *Applied Animal Ethology*. Vol. 10:5–17.

Ward, E. Association for Pet Obesity Prevention. August 2006. Unpublished data.

Grandjean, D, Paragon, BM. "Nutrition of racing and working dogs. Part I. Energy metabolism of dogs." *Compendium Continuing Education for Veterinarians*. 14(12):1608–1615.

Tipton, C. M., Carey, R. A., Eastin, W. C., and Erickson, H. H. "A submaximal test for dogs: evaluation of effects of training, detraining, and cage confinement." *Journal of Applied Physiology*. Aug 1974; 37: 271–275.

Hubrecht, RC, Seppel, JA and Poole, TB. "Correlates of pen size and housing conditions on the behavior of kenneled dogs." *Applied Animal Behavioral Science*. Vol. 34:365–383.

Tipton, C. M., Carey, R. A., Eastin, W. C., and Erickson, H. H. "A submaximal test for dogs: evaluation of effects of training, detraining, and cage confinement." *Journal of Applied Physiology*. Aug 1974; 37: 271–275.

Chan, CB, Spierenburg, M, Ihle, SL, Tudor-Locke, C. "Use of pedometers to measure physical activity in dogs." *Journal of the American Veterinary Medical Association*. Jun 15, 2005. Vol. 226(12); 2010–5.

CHAPTER 10 Rx 7: Track Your Progress

Lifestyle and Obesity. "How occasional indulgences shape a nation's waistline." *Thomson Medstat Research Brief*. July 2006.

"Dietary and physical activity behaviors among adults successful at weight loss maintenance." *International Journal of Behavioral Nutrition and Physical Activity*. July 2006, 3:17

Carciofi, AC et al. "A weight loss protocol and owners participation in the treatment of canine obesity." *Ciencia Rural*. Nov–Dec. 2005. Vol. 35 No. 6;1331–1338.

CHAPTER 11 Troubleshooting 101: Plateaus, Pestering, and Other Problems

Church, Timothy et al. "Changes in Weight, Waist Circumference and Compensatory Responses with Different Doses of Exercise among Sedentary, Overweight Postmenopausal Women." *PloS ONE* Vol. 4(2): e4515.

Sonneville, KR and Gortmaker, SL. "Total energy intake, adolescent discretionary behaviors and the energy gap." *International Journal of Obesity* (2008) 32, S19–S27

Lowe, Michael R., Butryn, Meghan L. "Hedonic hunger: A new dimension of appetite?" *Physiology & Behavior* July 2007. Vol. 91, Issue 4, 24;432–439; Proceedings from the 2006 Meeting of the Society for the Study of Ingestive Behavior.

Bergman, Richard et al. "Abdominal Obesity: Role in the Pathophysiology of Metabolic Disease and Cardiovascular Risk." *The American Journal of Medicine*. February 2007. Vol. 120, Issue 2, Supplement 1;S3–S8

CHAPTER 12 Weight Loss Supplements

Ishioka, K, Sagawa, M, Okumura, M, et al. "Treatment of obesity in dogs through increasing energy expenditure by mitochondrial uncoupling proteins." *Journal of Veterinary Internal Medicine.* 2004; 18:431

Ikeda, I, Sasaki, E, Yasunami, H, et al. "Digestion and lymphatic transport of eicosapentaenoic and docosahexaenoic acids given in the form of triacylglycerol, free acid and ethyl ester in rats." *Biochimica et Biophysica Acta (BBA)—Lipids and Lipid Metabolism* Volume 1259, Issue 3, 7 December 1995, Pages 297–304

Sunvold, GD, Tetrick, MA, Davenport, GM, et al. "Carnitine supplementation promotes weight loss and decreased adiposity in the canine." *Proceedings.* 23rd World Small Animal Veterinary Association 1998; 746

Maki KC, Davidson MH, Tsushima R, et al. "Consumption of diacylglycerol oil as part of a reduced-energy diet enhances loss of body weight and fat in comparison with consumption of a triacylglycerol control oil." *American Journal of Clinical Nutrition.* 2002 Dec;76(6):1230–6.

Umeda, T, Bauer, JE, Otsuji, K. "weigth loss effect of dietary diacylglycerol in obese dogs." *Journal of Animal Physiology and Animal Nutrition.* Vol. 90 (2006) 208–216

Bauer, John E., Nagaoka, Daisuke, Porterpan, Brandy, Bigley, Karen. "Postprandial Lipolytic Activities, Lipids, and Carbohydrate Metabolism Are Altered in Dogs Fed Diacylglycerol Meals Containing High- and Low-Glycemic-index Starches." *The Journal of Nutrition* 2006 Vol. 136 (no.7 Suppl)

Bierer, TL, Bui, LM. "High protein, low carbohydrate diets and not conjugated linoleic acid promote weight loss in overweight dogs." *Federation of American Societies for Experimental Biology Journal* 2004 Vol. 18:A874.

Jewell DE, Toll PW, Azain MJ, et al. "Fiber but not conjugated linoleic acid influences adiposity in dogs." *Veterinary Therapeutics* 2006 Vol. 7:78–85.

Pittler MH, Ernst E. "Dietary supplements for body-weight reduction: a systematic review." *American Journal of Clinical Nutrition.* 2004 Vol. 79:529–536.

Spears JW, Brown TT, Sunvold GD, et al. "Influence of chromium on glucose metabolism and insulin sensitivity." In: Reinhart GA, Carey DP, eds. *Recent advances in canine and feline nutrition.* Vol II. Wilmington, Ohio: Orange Frazer Press, 1998; pages 103–113.

Gross KL, Wedekind KJ, Kirk CA, et al. "Effect of dietary carnitine or chromium on weight loss and body composition of obese dogs." *Journal of Animal Science.* 1998 Vol. 76(suppl):175.

Gross KL, Wedekind KJ, Kirk CA, et al. Dietary chromium and carnitine supplementation does not affect glucose tolerance in obese dogs during weight loss." *Journal of Veterinary Internal Medicine* 2000 Vol. 14:345.

Kurzman ID, Panciera DL, Miller JB, et al. "The effect of dehydroepiandrosterone combined with a low-fat diet in spontaneously obese dogs: a clinical trial." *Obesity Research* 1998 Vol. 6:20–28.

MacEwen EG, Kuzman ID. "Obesity in the dog: role of the adrenal steroid dehydroepiandrosterone (DHEA)." *The Journal of Nutrition.* 1991 Vol. 121 (suppl 11):S51–S55.

Udani J, Singh B. "Blocking carbohydrate absorption and weight loss: a clinical trial using a proprietary fractionated white bean extract." *Alternative Therapies.* Jul/Aug 2007, Vol. 13, No. 4;32–37.

Bo-Linn GW, Santa Ana CA, Morawski SG, and Fordtran JS. "Starch blockers—their effect on calorie absorption from a high-starch meal." *The New England Journal of Medicine.* Vol. 307;1413–1416.

Carlson GL, Li BU, Bass P, and Olsen WA. "A bean alpha-amylase inhibitor formulation (starch blocker) is ineffective in man." *Science.* Vol. 219. No. 4583;393–395.

Leung LH. "Pantothenic acid as a weight-reducing agent: fasting without hunger, weakness and ketosis." *Medical Hypotheses* 1995;44:403–5.

Physicians' desk reference for herbal medicines. 2d ed. Montvale, N.J.: Medical Economics Company, 2000.

Sansone RA. "Complications of hazardous weight-loss methods." *American Family Physician.* 1984; 30:141–6.

Hielm-Björkman A, Reunanen V, Meri P, Tulam R-M. "Panax Ginseng in combination with brewers' yeast (Gerivet) as a stimulant for geriatric dogs: a controlled-randomized blinded study." *Journal of Veterinary Pharmacology and Therapeutics.* August 2007;30(4):295–304.

ConsumerLab.com. "Product Review: Fish Oil/Omega-3 Supplements and EPA/DHA Fortified Foods & Beverages." March 7, 2009. http://www.consumerlab.com/reviews/Omega-3_Fatty _Acids_EPA_and_DHA_from_Fish_Marine_Oils/omega3/

US Food and Drug Administration. "Survey Data on Lead in Women's and Children's Vitamins." August 2008. http://www.fda.gov/Food/FoodSafety/FoodContaminantsAdulteration/Metals/ Lead/ucm115941.htm

US Food and Drug Administration. "FDA Warns Consumers about Brazilian Diet Pills Found to Contain Active Drug Ingredients: Emagrece Sim and Herbathin Dietary Supplements May be Harmful." January 13, 2006. http://www.fda.gov/NewsEvents/Newsroom/PressAnnounce ments/2006/ucm108578.htm

ConsumerLab.com. "Consumerlab.com Finds Fifty Fish Oil Supplements Free Of Contaminants In Fish: New Report Helps Consumers Choose Among Pills, Liquids, Foods and Beverages with Omega-3 Fatty Acids (EPA and DHA)." August 5, 2008. http://www.consumerlab.com/news/ Omega-3_Fatty_Acids_EPA_and_DHA_from_Fish_Marine_Oils/08_05_2008/

ConsumerLab.com. "Consumerlab.Com Testing Of Alpha Lipoic Acid Supplements From Japan Finds No Ingredient In One Product; Most Others Meet Claims: Japanese Consumers Urged to Research Product Quality." August 31, 2005. http://www.consumerlab.com/news/Japanese_ Alpha_Lipoic_Acid_Supplements/08_31_2005/

"Slentrol (Dirlotapide) "First to Know." Pfizer Animal Health. 2007.

CHAPTER 13 When Obesity Goes Unchecked: The Consequences of Excess Weight

McCay C. M., Crowell Mary F. "Prolonging the Life Span." *The Scientific Monthly.* Nov 1934. Vol. 39, No. 5;405–414.

Kealy, Richard D., Lawler, Dennis F., Ballam, Joan M., Mantz, Sandra L., et al. "Effects of diet restriction on life span and age-related changes in dogs." *Journal of the American Veterinary Medical Association.* May 1, 2002, Vol. 220, No. 9;1315–1320.

Lawler, Dennis F., Evans, Richard H., Larson, Brian T., et al. "Influence of lifetime food restriction on causes, time, and predictors of death in dogs." *Journal of the American Veterinary Medical Association.* January 15, 2005, Vol. 226, No. 2;225–231.

Venable, Rachel O., Stoker, Aaron M., Cook, Cristi R., et al. "Examination of synovial fluid hyaluronan quantity and quality in stifle joints of dogs with osteoarthritis." *American Journal of Veterinary Research.* December 2008, Vol. 69, No. 12;1569–1573.

Keaney, Jr. John F., Larson, Martin G., Vasan, Ramachandran S., Wilson, Peter W.F., et al. "Obesity and Systemic Oxidative Stress. Clinical Correlates of Oxidative Stress in The Framingham Study." *Arteriosclerosis, Thrombosis, and Vascular Biology.* 2003 Vol. 23;434–439.

Cline MG, Lauren, S, Cox, S, Bartges, JW. "The relationship between obesity and markers of oxidative stress in dogs" *Journal of Animal Physiology and Animal Nutrition.* Vol. 93 Issue 2:141–142.

Larson, BT, Lawler, DF, Spitznagel, Jr., EL and Kealy, RD. "Improved Glucose Tolerance with Lifetime Diet Restriction Favorably Affects Disease and Survival in Dogs." *The Journal of Nutrition.* 133 (9):2887–92.

Kooistra,HS, Galac, S, Buijtels, JJCWM, Meij, BP "Endocrine diseases in animals." *Hormone Research.* January 2009;71 Suppl 1(0):144–7.

Rand, Jacquie S., et al. "Canine and Feline Diabetes Mellitus: Nature or Nurture?" *The Journal of Nutrition.* August 2004. 134:2072S–2080S.

Catchpole, B, Ristic, JM, Fleeman, LM, Davison, LJ. "Canine diabetes mellitus: can old dogs teach us new tricks?" *Diabetologia.* October 2005;48(10):1948–56.

Ellmerer, Martin et al. "Reduced access to insulin-sensitive tissues in dogs with obesity secondary to increased fat intake." *Diabetes.* June 2006;55(6):1769–75.

Guptill, L, Glickman, L, Glickman, N. "Time trends and risk factors for diabetes mellitus in dogs: analysis of veterinary medical data base records (1970–1999)." *The Veterinary Journal.* May 2003;165(3):240–7.

DeFronzo, RA and Ferrannini, E. "Insulin resistance. A multifaceted syndrome responsible for NIDDM, obesity, hypertension, dyslipidemia, and atherosclerotic cardiovascular disease." *Diabetes Care.* March 1991 vol. 14 no. 3;173–194.

Bloomgarden, Zachary T. "Obesity, Hypertension, and Insulin Resistance." *Diabetes Care.* November 2002 vol. 25 no. 11;2088–2097.

Craig, BW, Garthwaite, SM and Holloszy, JO. "Adipocyte insulin resistance: effects of aging, obesity, exercise, and food restriction." *Journal of Applied Physiology.* Vol 62, Issue 1;95–100.

Rocchini, AP, Mao, HZ. "Clonidine Prevents Insulin Resistance and Hypertension in Obese Dogs." *Hypertension* 1999;33;548–553.

FJ Martinez, RA Rizza and JC Romero. "High-fructose feeding elicits insulin resistance, hyperinsulinism, and hypertension in normal mongrel dogs." *Hypertension.* 1994. Vol. 23;456–463.

JE Hall, MW Brands, WN Dixon, and MJ Smith Jr. "Obesity-induced hypertension. Renal function and systemic hemodynamics." *Hypertension.* 1993; 22:292–299.

Philip-Couderc P, Smih F, Pelat M, Vidal C, et al. "Cardiac transcriptome analysis in obesity-related hypertension." *Hypertension.* Mar 2003. Vol. 41(3);414–21.

Bravo, PE, Morse, S, Borne, DM, et al. "Leptin and Hypertension in Obesity." *Vascular Health Risk Management.* June 2006. Vol. 2(2);163–169.

Jeusette, IC, Lhoest, ET, Istasse, LP, and Diez, MO. "Influence of obesity on plasma lipid and lipoprotein concentrations in dogs." *American Journal of Veterinary Research.* Jan 2005. Vol. 66(1);81–6.

Caballero, AE. "Endothelial Dysfunction in Obesity and Insulin Resistance: A Road to Diabetes and Heart Disease." *Obesity Research.* Vol. 11: 1278–1289.

Bach, JF, Rozanski, EA, Bedenice, D, et al. "Association of expiratory airway dysfunction with marked obesity in healthy adult dogs." *American Journal of Veterinary Research.* Jun 2007. Vol. 68(6);670–5.

Wilke, VL, Robinson, DA, Evans, RB, et al. "Estimate of the annual economic impact of treatment of cranial cruciate ligament injury in dogs in the United States." *Journal of the American Veterinary Medical Association.* November 15, 2005. Vol 227, No. 10;1604–07.

Veterinary Pet Insurance. "Veterinary Pet Insurance Reveals Most Expensive Pet Conditions: Pets of All Ages Susceptible to Costly Accidents and Illnesses." Jan. 14, 2008. http://press.petinsurance.com/pressroom/236.aspx

Alonso-Galicia, M, Dwyer, TM, Herrera, GA, Hall, JE. "Increased Hyaluronic Acid in the Inner Renal Medulla of Obese Dogs." *Hypertension.* 1995. Vol. 25;888–892.

Rahmouni, K, Correia, M, Haynes, WG, Mar, AL. "Obesity-Associated Hypertension: New Insights Into Mechanisms." *Hypertension.* 2005. Vol. 45;9–14.

Gu, Jian-Wei et al. "Cytokine gene expression profiles in kidney medulla and cortex of obese hypertensive dogs." *Kidney International.* 2004. Vol. 66, 713–721.

Aneja, A, et al. "Hypertension and Obesity." *Recent Progress in Hormone Research.* 2004. Vol. 59(1);169–205.

Henegar, JR, Bigler, SA et al. "Functional and Structural Changes in the Kidney in the Early Stages of Obesity." *Journal of the American Society of Nephrology.* 2001. Vol. 12;1211–1217.

Hall, JE, Brands, MW, Dixon, WN and Smith, MJ. "Obesity-induced hypertension. Renal function and systemic hemodynamics." *Hypertension*, Vol 22, 292–299.

Rocchini Albert P., Moorehead, Catherine, Wentz, Elliot; and Deremer, Susan. "Obesity-Induced Hypertension in the Dog." Hypertension. Vol 9 (Suppl III) III-64-68.

Rocchini, AP, Moorehead, CP, DeRemer, S and Bondie, D. "Pathogenesis of weight-related changes in blood pressure in dogs." *Hypertension.* 1989;13:922–928.

Klassen, A, Bahner, U, Sebekova, K, and Heidland, A. "The importance of overweight and obesity for the development and progression of renal diseases." *Deutsche medizinische Wochenschrift.* March 2004;129(11):579–82.

National Cancer Institute. "Obesity and Cancer: Questions and Answers: Fact Sheet." March 16, 2004. http://www.cancer.gov/cancertopics/factsheet/Risk/obesity

Vainio H, Bianchini F. IARC handbooks of cancer prevention. Volume 6: Weight control and physical activity. Lyon, France: IARC Press, 2002.

Hursting, Stephen D., Nunez, Nomeli P., Varticovski, Lyuba, and Vinson, Charles. "The Obesity-Cancer Link: Lessons Learned from a Fatless Mouse." *Cancer Research.* 2007 67: 2391–2393.

Hayashidani, Hideki et al. "Quantitative Survey on Relation between Obesity and Disease in Pet Dogs: Obesity Increases Risk of Diseases Two-fold." Kao Company correspondence. Published online March 26, 2009. http://www.kao.com/jp/en/corp_news/2009/20090326_001.html?

Agarwal, Sanjay K., Vogel, Klara, Weitsman, Stacy R., and Magoffin, Denis A. "Leptin Antagonizes the Insulin-Like Growth Factor-I Augmentation of Steroidogenesis in Granulosa and Theca Cells of the Human Ovary." *The Journal of Clinical Endocrinology & Metabolism.* Vol. 84, No. 3:1072–76.

Robker, Rebecca L. et al. "Obese Women Exhibit Differences in Ovarian Metabolites, Hormones, and Gene Expression Compared with Moderate-Weight Women." *The Journal of Clinical Endocrinology & Metabolism.* Vol. 94, No. 5 1533–1540.

Bamgbade, Nafiu et al. "Postoperative complications in obese and nonobese patients," *World Journal of Surgery.* March 2007, Vol. 31, 556—560.

German, AJ. "Complications of Overnutrition in Companion Animals." *Clinician's Brief.* March 2008; 11–14.

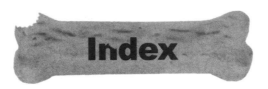

Index

Page numbers followed by an *f* or *t* indicate figures or tables.

About the Author

DR. ERNEST WARD, DVM, or "Dr. Ernie," is a practicing veterinarian who is dedicated to helping pets and their humans live healthier lives. He appears regularly on the *Rachael Ray Show*, and has been featured on Animal Planet, NBC *Nightly News*, the *Today Show* and CNN. He has authored and contributed to over fifty-five veterinary journal articles in North America, England, Canada, Japan, and China, and has published three books and three veterinary training videos. He lectures extensively in the United States, Canada, Europe, and China, and was awarded the Speaker of the Year award from the North American Veterinary Conference in 2004. An athlete himself, he is an avid racer, certified personal trainer, triathlon coach, and Ironman; he competed in the inaugural Ford Ironman 70.3 World Championships and the 2008 Escape from Alcatraz triathlon. Visit his websites: www.DrErnieWard.com, and www.PetObesityPrevention.com, and www.ChowHoundsBook.com.

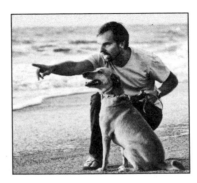